THE ONE WAY DIET

The pathway to weight loss

Toni Pike

Text copyright © 2017 Toni Pike
Cover design © 2017 Toni Pike
All Rights Reserved

All Rights Reserved. No part of this book may be used or reproduced in any manner whatsoever without written permission, except in the case of brief quotations embodied in articles and reviews about the book.

First published in December 2017 – *Kindle Edition.*

This is the first paperback edition: December 2017

ISBN: 9781973569251

www.tonipike.com

Disclaimer
This book does not contain any medical advice.
This is a personal story, and should not be seen as professional advice.
Results may vary because the causes of obesity and other factors vary from person to person. No individual results should be seen as typical.
The information in this book has not been evaluated by the Food and Drug Administration and is not intended in any way as a substitute for professional medical advice, diagnosis or treatment. Always seek the advice of your physician or other qualified health care provider regarding any questions you may have about any medical condition or treatment, and any weight loss program. Before you undertake any new health care regimen, always seek advice from your physician or other qualified health care provider. Never disregard professional medical advice or delay seeking it because of something you read in this book.

About the Author

Toni Pike is an Australian who loves to travel the world doing research for her thrillers. As well as *The Jotham Fletcher Mystery Thriller Series*, she has a book of travel tips and enjoys sharing travel photos on Instagram: @authorlovestravel. You can also find her at tonipike.com.

Other works
The Jotham Fletcher Mystery Thriller Series
Book 1: THE MAGUS COVENANT
Book 2: THE ROCK OF MAGUS
Book 3: THE MAGUS EPIPHANY

HAPPY TRAVELS 101 is a book of travel tips: *Don't leave home without these cruise, flight, safety, packing and sightseeing tips*

Table of Contents

INTRODUCTION

Are you searching for the pathway to weight loss?

This is a no-nonsense guide to finding the slender person you dream about, with simple advice on how to lose weight by focusing on your goals. THE ONE WAY DIET is not just a healthy eating plan, but is also about coping with every aspect of your weight loss journey.

People often say to me now that I'm lucky because I don't have to worry about my weight. How wrong they are! Five years ago, I lost more than thirty kilograms after a lifetime of weight problems. Every day since then, I make the lifestyle choice to stay slim.

It's called THE ONE WAY DIET because when I followed this method, my weight moved in one direction only until I reached my goal weight of sixty kilograms.

I'm giving you the benefit of my personal experience about weight loss, but there are no wild theories in this book. All you will find here is useful information and powerful inspiration.

You'll find out why most people gain weight and what I believe is the most effective way to lose it. Discover how to keep yourself motivated and how to cope with the challenges of everyday life. Be prepared for each stage of your weight loss journey and learn how to avoid a weight loss plateau.

Always seek the advice of your doctor before starting a weight loss program, and always follow their advice. I'm not a qualified health professional, but I do have a science degree and have worked in health-related fields.

If your dream is to lose weight, then this book will help to give you the tools that you need to succeed.

You have nothing to lose but your excess weight, and everything to gain.

Measurements

I use British spelling because I live in Australia, and like to use kilograms and calories when talking about weight loss.

To help convert measurements, here is a simple table:

1 pound = 0.45 kilograms

1 kilogram = 2.2 pounds

100 grams = 3.5 ounces or 0.22 pounds
1 pound = 454 grams
60 kilograms = 132 pounds
100 kilograms = 220 pounds
1 inch = 2.54 centimetres
1 centimetre = 0.39 inches
100 calories = 418.4 kilojoules
1,200 calories = 5,020 kilojoules
1,500 calories = 6,276 kilojoules

CHAPTER 1: MY WEIGHT LOSS STORY

My own history of weight loss and gain

The time has come for you to travel on a very special journey to find that slender person that you've always dreamed about. It's a long, slow journey with challenges along the way. But it will be full of wonderful moments and you will never regret it.

I was that fat kid in class, the one who looked twice as large as all the other children, and my weight has cycled up and down since then with all the wild abandon of a rollercoaster. A graph of my weight from birth would keep a brilliant team of mathematicians entertained for a long time. I have been there, done that, then been there and done it again.

But five years ago, everything changed. I completed a weight loss journey using the key principles that I outline in this book and discovered the slender person that I was always meant to be. I've remained slim since them, and I'm determined to remain slim for the rest of my life.

You might wonder why I decided to write a book about weight loss, or why I would claim to have both experience and knowledge of the subject. That's why I want to share with you a little about my past, talk about my experience with weight loss and gain, and tell you about my education.

Here is a diary excerpt from six years ago, when I was overweight.

Oh Dear, Dear Diary

In 2002 I looked and felt wonderful after losing twenty kilos and starting a new job in the public service. Now, ten years later, I've gained weight, lost some, gained some more and now my weight is steadily on the rise. Last week, I saw an old family movie of me at my best. It made me feel very sad. If only I could be like that again! If only I could go to sleep, and when I woke up, there was thin me back again! Where did it all go so wrong?

Does my diary excerpt sound at all familiar? If practice makes perfect and skill and knowledge is gained by doing things over and over, then I'm certainly an expert on weight loss and almost a genius at weight gain. The dictionary defines an expert as someone with knowledge and experience. I do have some scientific and medical knowledge and I have plenty of experience with weight loss, even more with weight gain, and a long history of reading good, reliable, scientifically based information about diets and nutrition.

My vast experience with weight loss and gain began when I was a baby.

My mother could not produce enough breast milk, so I was fed with a mixture made from condensed milk. Can you believe it? In those days there were no baby formulas and, as you know, condensed milk is packed with sugar. I'm sure that didn't help my fat cells get off to a good start, although it wasn't until third, fourth and fifth grade that I was overweight. We didn't know much about good nutrition. There was always a supply of chocolate biscuits and a wide variety of other fattening treats available at home, which certainly didn't help me.

In those days there were not as many overweight children as there are now, so I was the only child in my class who wasn't skinny. I would look enviously at all my friends with their thin little bodies. Of course there was plenty of name-calling, but that doesn't matter now.

Somehow, I slimmed down for sixth grade, had a wonderful year and was slender throughout high school. During university I gained the odd kilo or two, but managed to lose it by occasional dieting.

I married an Air Force officer when I was twenty-five, enjoyed a posting to England during our first year of marriage and had two beautiful children in the next few years. There was plenty of weight gain during my first pregnancy and even more during my second. But I managed to slim down after both pregnancies by following a sensible diet.

In 1989 we were lucky enough to be posted to Washington D.C. in America, where we had a wonderful three years. After that, we returned to Australia and now live in Canberra.

I suppose it was 1990 when my weight started to creep slowly upwards like a heavily laden train climbing a hill. By the time we were living in Melbourne in 1993, I was decidedly overweight. By the time we moved to Canberra in 1998, I weighed more than ninety kilos. And I had spent my thirties, perhaps the best years of my life, being overweight.

I would not say that I was binge eater. I didn't eat enormous amounts, but added a variety of treats to my menu all day and ate much more than I needed. My biggest downfall was chocolate. There was a regular supply on hand and it never stayed in the cupboard for long.

In 2001, I finally started a sensible diet, learnt how to cook the low-fat way, and stayed with it until I reached the healthy weight for my height of 69 kilos. I'm average height, about 166 centimetres tall. It took me well over a year to lose that weight, and at the start of 2002 I began a new career with the public service. I was so happy and proud! It was wonderful to be slim and to feel slim, to fit into size twelve clothes and buy whatever I wanted in fashion stores. When I looked down at my body, it wasn't too fat! It was exhilarating to feel like a normal person.

Slowly, though, my weight started to creep up again, with just a few extra things to eat, a morning tea here, a candy bar there, and making excuses for myself that I needed this or that to eat to get through the day. My weight rose to about 90 kilos, then came down again, and climbed back to about 85 kilos. I lost a few kilos, but then the weight started that upward rise once more.

In 2009, with our children grown up, we went on our first ocean cruise and had a fantastic time. Since then, we've taken a cruise nearly every year, exploring the world and having fun. But two weeks a year of eating too much delicious food for breakfast, lunch and dinner helped to pile on the weight.

Once in the habit of eating too much, it's easy to say yes to every eating opportunity that presents itself. At the start of 2012, I weighed more than ninety kilos.

That's when I decided to start a very special journey that has changed my life. As you see, I can claim to be an expert on weight gain and weight loss because of my vast experience. I want to share with you my understanding and my very simple theories about the difficult challenge of losing weight. And along the way, I hope that you'll find that slender person you were meant to be.

My career and education

I'm not a qualified health professional. You must see a doctor or other qualified health professional before embarking on any weight loss program. Always take their advice, and do not hesitate to seek their guidance with any issues you may have. Never take any advice from this book, except under their guidance.

I do, however, have a scientific background, and was educated in Australia. I have a Bachelor of Veterinary Science degree and also a Postgraduate Diploma in Education. I've worked for the Australian government in health-related fields, and spent many years as a high school science teacher while my children were growing up. That has given some awareness of health and nutrition, and a sound respect for the medical profession. I believe in placing my faith in scientific knowledge. I've also worked with the manufacture of veterinary medicines and know all the effort that goes into the manufacture of registered medicines.

This guide provides sensible advice

I strongly believe in a well-balanced, nutritious diet that includes all the major food groups. And I believe in doing everything in moderation, in small steps.

So if you want a crazy, extreme diet then don't read any further. I won't be advising you to eat a bucket of spinach a day, or cleanse a major organ, or go on regular fasting rituals. I won't tell you to exercise for four hours a day, or insist that you can't lose weight unless you jog ten kilometres up and down a hill every morning. I won't claim to have invented some wondrous new way to lose weight, or know something that nobody else knows.

I'll only be talking about real food, not protein shakes, diet biscuits or any other substitutes. I believe in eating wholesome, healthy food as long as we are on planet Earth and not trying to survive in a space capsule.

The next chapter talks about that very special moment when we finally decide to embark on a weight loss journey. It's so important for you to value that moment and never look back.

CHAPTER 2: THE MOMENT YOU DECIDE TO LOSE WEIGHT

The moment of clarity

The moment of clarity is the most mysterious and extraordinary part of losing weight. It comes in one lucid moment before anyone starts to follow a weight loss program. No one, not even the person losing weight, can explain why suddenly, after years of longing and setting goals they never met, everything changes. Suddenly they start the diet that changes their life.

I call it the moment of clarity because it's a magic moment when the fog in our mind lifts and our purpose is instantly clear.

Just pretend for a moment that you want to go on a holiday. Not just a few days by the beach, but an overseas trip that you've been thinking about for a long time. You've had a vague idea in your mind that you'd love to see a certain part of the world. Many of us, I'm sure, have a dream or two like that in our heads. If you've already travelled all over the world, think about the time before that started and the places that were top of your list.

When and how is it that we start to think of seeing a certain part of the world? When and how do we decide that we'd love to see Scandinavia or Asia or spend a month in Italy? Did that start years ago, perhaps even when we were a child? I know when I was a child I always dreamed of visiting the USA, and later I longed to visit Europe. Other people might decide that they want to trek through the Himalayas or climb Mt Kilimanjaro. You definitely won't see me there! We all have different travel dreams, and while many people these days are able to travel, for many others it remains a dream for the future.

When is it that we actually start to take action to make those dreams a reality? Sometimes, people start planning a trip years in advance while others will leave it to the last minute. There's always a moment, though, when the dreams change and start to become real plans instead of a thought bubble.

It's exactly the same with your weight loss journey. Before you start to plan your weight loss you need to have that wonderful dream about being thinner. The bridge between those two things is that magical moment of clarity.

Here is a diary excerpt from just before my moment of clarity. Do you think that I sound like I'm ready to take on the challenge?

Dear Diary,

Once again, I find myself weighing 94 kilos. Many of the clothes I wore a year ago don't fit me any more, or are very tight. Have I been in denial? I don't think so. I've been aware every second of the day that my body was fat, that my legs are huge, and that so many others I see around me at work are slender and look fantastic in their cute little dresses. How I'd love to be like that!

Why is that we take so long to reach that moment, and what makes us suddenly leap across that chasm?

Those goals we never met

People will spend years wishing they could lose weight. There may have been all sorts of reasons to motivate them into weight loss, and many goals that they wanted to achieve. They might want to look better for their next holiday, a wedding or a party, or even lose weight to improve their health. There might have been cruel comments from other people, or they had an awful time trying to shop for clothes that wouldn't fit properly. And of course they had well-meaning advice from doctors, friends or family.

Every one of those goals was the perfect motivating factor. But did it cause them to reach that moment of clarity? No, of course it didn't. And then suddenly there is one more moment, one more factor and the decision is made, and the journey begun.

I found that the most confronting moment of all was trying on clothes in a fashion store. There is something about those mirrors in a fitting room that makes you look twice as fat. Maybe it's because you're standing so close to the mirror dressed in underwear, with another mirror right behind you, so you get the full three dimensional picture. Surely that would make a person want to lose weight? Of course it should, but somehow that never brought me to my moment of clarity. All it did was make me upset.

For years I've set goal after goal and watched them pass me by, often gaining weight instead of losing it and starting diets that lasted less than a day. There have been a couple of family weddings and several vacations that I planned far in advance and that could have motivated me to lose weight. I would have loved to lose weight for that summer holiday in Fiji so that I wouldn't look like a beached whale in my swimming costume. But sometimes, those special events looming in the future can feel like a threat, and that feeling of intimidation can stop us sticking to our diet.

I remember my daughter's twenty-first birthday party. We gave her a wonderful party at the local golf club with dinner for about fifty guests, and as always she looked beautiful and slender. But I had managed to gain masses of weight in the months leading up to the party, and then left buying an outfit until the last minute. Because it was between seasons, there was barely anything left in the stores that would fit me. I wore a ghastly dress and was sure I looked terrible, even though we all had a wonderful time. I felt like I had let my family down.

Why is it that despite wanting to lose weight, we don't start that diet? Or perhaps we start it, and it only lasts a few days or even less. Is it lack of motivation or willpower? Are we greedy or gluttonous, and won't deprive ourselves of excessive food consumption? Or are we simply too lazy to get ourselves motivated?

No, of course not! If you believe those things, then you've succumbed to the same fat discrimination that pervades the world. You're not weak, stupid, out of control or unable to function as a normal human being. You're simply a very normal person who hasn't yet experienced that moment of clarity, despite your dreams of losing weight.

Comments from other people

I've been very fortunate. My husband and family never mentioned my weight gain and never made snide remarks. But for many people, comments from other people can become a major concern that ruins their self-confidence.

Our doctors are interested primarily in our health care and have every right to tell us that we ought to lose weight. For some people, that could be the moment of clarity that is needed. There could even be a health scare: a current one or the promise of health problems in the future.

The comments that never bring that moment of clarity are nasty comments, snide remarks, so-called humorous remarks, and nagging from friends and relatives. I often wonder why people seem to think that it's their duty to comment on a person's weight gain. Do they truly think we haven't noticed? That it will come as some sort of newsflash that we need to act on?

Usually we know that our family and friends are just trying to help, even if they see how upset it makes us. But the comments are unnecessary and destructive for two very good reasons.

The first reason is that we already know we're overweight, much better than anyone else. In fact, if you're anything like me, you think about it constantly. You have to live with seeing yourself in the mirror, and trying on those clothes that don't fit, or are becoming too tight. We've seen ourselves in photographs with family and friends, looking twice as wide as everyone else, smiling at the camera with a round face and double chin. No comment will tell us anything new.

The second reason is that all those comments will never result in the desired effect of starting someone on the path to weight loss. They only have the negative effect of making us feel more hopeless and depressed about our weight gain. And that only leads to more overeating.

You would think that those comments should jolt us into action. Sometimes one chance remark can bring us closer to the moment of clarity. But it's not because of the comments that we reach that moment. It's because we already knew that we needed to lose weight and have decided, all by ourselves, to make that first step.

The trigger moment before our brains light up

The moment of clarity has two stages. First, there is the trigger moment when something happens, big or small.

We've all heard of the trigger on a gun. We pull the trigger, and then fire the gun. And until that trigger is pulled, the gun will not fire a single shot. But after the trigger is pulled, it's ready, aim, fire! It's exactly the same with us. Just like that, we have a trigger moment and then a moment of clarity, and we're off! Changing our life forever!

What could be a trigger moment? It can be big or small, and it can be something that has already happened to us dozens or hundreds of times before. You could try on a favourite outfit and find that it's too tight, or hear a chance remark, or start to plan a vacation and realise that you might have enough time to lose that weight. You could see somebody in the street and wish that you could look like them. Or you could simply look at your calendar or start a new year and decide that the time has come. Slowly and carefully, you pull that trigger in your mind.

The real trigger is not the event that happened to you. The trigger is a thought process in your head, the reaction you have to that special moment. After that, you flick a switch in your mind and suddenly turn on a light bulb in your brain.

The light bulb moment when we decide to lose weight

The light bulb moment is the second stage in the moment of clarity.

I once worked in a new building where the lights automatically switched off several times a day. That made my small office very dark, so I had to walk to the door and press the light switch. Instantly, there was bright light.

Our brains are just like that. First there's a trigger moment that sets off all sorts of sparks and interconnections inside our head. Then we press the switch, and have light! We emerge from the darkness.

The human brain is a very complex piece of machinery, with millions of interconnections. Scientists have only started to understand it, and when you combine all that with our heart and soul, you can see why no one can really explain what makes us suddenly decide to do something.

How do you know that you've reached that moment of clarity and turned on a light bulb in your brain? To tell the truth, that very special moment might be over so quickly, you don't realise that it's happened. You'll remember the trigger moment, but the light bulb moment is hard to recall.

The truth is that you don't have to know exactly when it happened, or why. You'll know that it's happened, though, because in the next moment, you're starting to make plans and imagine yourself being slim.

CHAPTER 3: THE KEY INGREDIENTS TO WEIGHT LOSS

The secret to weight loss

Just imagine a baker who's keen to bake a cake. He's well qualified and experienced, with a great reputation. He has excellent equipment, with a high quality oven, cake tin and utensils. But when he starts to make the cake, he finds that he doesn't have any flour. He doesn't even have any eggs. All he has is his bare hands and some butter, sugar and vanilla essence. There's no way that he can make a cake with only those items. He mumbles to himself that he's missing the key ingredients for his masterpiece.

He goes to the grocery store and buys some flour and eggs, then starts cooking and succeeds in making a beautiful cake. Do you see how important those key ingredients were? He knew that he wanted to make a cake, he had the recipe and all the skills to do it, but without the right key ingredients it would never happen.

Now I want to share a special secret with you, because you're going to learn what I believe is the secret to losing weight. I'm not going to tell you that you need diet and exercise, a special magic potion, or a powdered formula created by a mysterious guru from a foreign country. The real secret to losing weight isn't any of those things, because it lies deep within your heart and mind.

The secret is that you need the four key ingredients to weight loss.

If you're willing to learn about them and use them correctly, then you can become that slender person of your dreams. The whole world will see it and you'll receive more compliments than you ever thought possible.

When you see a packet of flour, a canister of sugar and a tray of eggs on the kitchen bench, is it hard to imagine a cake? After an hour you'll create a cake, but you need to have the key ingredients or it would be impossible.

I believe that the four key ingredients to weight loss are belief, knowledge, plans and action. This book is about those four key ingredients, and in this chapter I want to outline them briefly. You can't buy them at the local supermarket or a pharmacy, or even a hardware store. We're not talking about a cake. The first place to look for them is deep within your heart and mind, and you can begin to understand them by being willing to learn about them.

Key Ingredient Number One: Belief

The first key ingredient that you need for weight loss is belief. The first step to making something happen is to be convinced that it's possible. It doesn't matter if you don't know how you will make it happen yet. You will become the slender you. Can you believe it, or is that too difficult to imagine?

First, think about the very special person that you are now. Do you feel sometimes as if there's a slender person inside you, screaming to get out? We all feel like a thin, beautiful human being deep inside. That's because there truly is a slender person there, that you've kept hidden for far too long.

In the next chapter, you're going to think about what your life would be like if you were slender right now, and if you'd always been slender. The person you'll be thinking about will be identical to you, except for the amount of fat in their body.

Can you imagine that person right now, and do you wish that you could be like them? Do you want to become that person, or does that just seem unattainable?

The truth is that the task isn't impossible. That person just made a few different choices. In every other way, they're the same as you. And I'm here to assure you that you can become that slender person you long to be – so long as you believe that it's possible.

That's the first key ingredient to weight loss. You must believe with all your heart that you can become that slender person. Picture them in your mind. That will be your goal, and something that will always motivate you.

But do you still have doubts? In that case, you need to focus on finding just the smallest kernel of belief and making it grow until you believe with all your heart that you can be slim.

Some people have gained weight only in the last few years. It will be easy for them to imagine being slim, and they might have some lovely photographs from the past to help them have faith in themselves that they can be that person again. The camera doesn't lie, as we all know. Belief for them will not be too difficult.

Some other people will have a more difficult challenge, because they've been overweight all their lives and might find it hard to imagine how they would look or feel. They're the ones who need to search in their heart and latch on tightly to every morsel of belief that they can muster.

If you have the key ingredient of belief, if you believe that you can become that slender person of your dreams, then you've taken the very first step on your weight loss journey.

Key Ingredient Number Two: Knowledge

The second key ingredient that you need for weight loss is knowledge. You need to learn how to lose weight.

Imagine a hairdresser who wants to cut and style your hair. They have a sharp pair of scissors, and they're very keen to do the job. But that alone won't help them to create an amazing hairstyle. They also need the skill that they've gained through training and study. That knowledge is the key ingredient that separates a great hairdresser from a person in the street.

You need to learn about healthy eating, exercise, and everything else that will help you complete your weight loss journey. You need to master those skills before you get started. Otherwise, you won't know how to successfully lose weight.

Most of this book is designed to give you some basic knowledge about healthy, sensible weight loss. When you finish reading it, you'll have enough knowledge to get started on a weight loss program.

Where else can you learn how to lose weight? The very best source of knowledge is your own doctor or another qualified health professional that your doctor recommends. It's essential to speak to your doctor before you embark on a weight loss program, and also to talk to them if you have any health issues.

I wouldn't be surprised if you're feeling a bit confused about how to lose weight. There's so much information about weight loss available in books, on the Internet, in magazines and on television. Even your best friends are on the latest extreme diet, and they are normally so sensible, aren't they?

By gaining the key ingredient of knowledge, you'll be better able to judge for yourself whether information about weight loss is good or bad. If the information tells you to take a magic formula or supplement, or exercise for hours every day, or cut out several food groups, then you can put it in the bad category. Also in the bad category are promises of losing a large amount of weight in a small amount of time. Read the fine print: you'll see a different promise there.

If the information tells you to have a sensible diet that includes all the food groups, and to have a moderate amount of exercise, then you can put it in the good category.

Always ask your doctor for their opinion about any weight loss information, and follow their advice.

Once you have the key ingredient of knowledge and learn how to lose weight, then you've taken the second step on your weight loss journey.

Key Ingredient Number Three: A Master Plan

The third key ingredient that you need is a master plan. You believe that you can become slender and you've gained some knowledge. You've learnt what you need to do in order to lose weight. It's one of your dreams, isn't it? And unlike some dreams, you know that you really can achieve it.

But now you need to turn your dream into a master plan. You need to have a plan for your weight loss journey, and after you've learnt how to lose weight, you can start to write that plan.

Towards the end of this book, you'll learn how to design a master plan for your weight loss journey. You'll use it to record your progress, and it will include your eating plan, exercise program, shopping, cooking, and how to stay motivated.

Some of you will be very well organised people, always writing lists and arranging your life. Planning will come easily to you and seem like the sensible thing to do.

Others will be putting their hands up in the air, saying "Stop right there – I never plan anything. I love to get out of bed and live from moment to moment." Or perhaps you feel that your life is always disorganised and chaotic, your desk is littered with paper, and that is just the way you are.

Don't worry if you feel like that. It's easy to design a master plan for your weight loss journey. When you realise the key role it plays in keeping you motivated, and you write down your first weight loss measurement, then you'll become more enthusiastic about it.

If you have the key ingredient of a master plan, then you've already taken the third step on your weight loss journey.

Key Ingredient Number Four: Action

The fourth key ingredient that you need for weight loss is action. You need to turn your dreams into a plan and then take action to implement your plan.

You believe that you can become the slender you, you've learnt what you have to do and you've turned your dream into a master plan. You can look at your plan and admire it, and you can desperately long to lose weight. But it won't happen until you take action take action and implement your plan.

That sounds so simple, so logical that you must wonder why I'm bothering to say it. Of course we have to start doing something in order to lose weight. But if you read about my story and think about your own then you'll realise why it's so important.

That initial step of taking action to start a weight loss program is incredibly difficult for most of us, almost like a mountain that we can't climb. And yet, at the same time, it's incredibly easy. In Chapter 2, I talked about that magic moment when we take a step into the unknown.

The incredible thing is that you can do it. All you have to do is take that initial step of putting your master plan into action. It's much easier than staying overweight. It isn't like climbing a mountain or rowing single-handed across the Pacific Ocean. Those things are as difficult as they sound.

If you start to carry out your plan to lose weight, then you have discovered the key ingredient of taking action. You have taken the fourth step on your weight loss journey and already you have reached the summit because the rest will be downhill.

Remember the secret to losing weight? *You can become the slender person of your dreams, and the key ingredients that you need are belief, knowledge, plans and action.*

Now - are you ready to find out more?

The next chapter is about the key ingredient of belief: imagining the slender you and believing that you can become that person.

Chapters 5 – 25 are about the key ingredient of knowledge. Those chapters are like a training manual, showing you how to lose weight and cope with every aspect of your weight loss journey.

Chapter 26 is about the key ingredient of a master plan, and shows you how to write your own master plan for your weight loss journey.

Chapter 27 is about the key ingredient of action, and the importance of taking action to follow your plan until you reach your goal weight.

CHAPTER 4: BELIEVE IN THE SLENDER YOU

Believe that you can become slim

The first key ingredient to losing weight is to believe that you can become the slender person of your dreams. The best way to do that is to visualise what you life would be like if you were slender right now.

Once you've done that, you then have a goal. You will have a mental picture of how you will look and feel when you reach your target weight. Every day, that will motivate you to continue your weight loss journey and keep following the One Way Diet.

Imagine if there was a slender you

Imagine if there was a slender you, living in a world exactly like yours. The person that I want you to imagine is almost identical to the real you. They have all your thoughts and feelings, the same friends and family, the same house, the same heart, head and soul.

But that is where the similarity ends because this slender person has never been overweight. They've never suffered from all the difficulties that come along with being fat, and they've never had to suffer from discrimination because of their weight.

Imagine what your life might be like if that slender person was you. You jump out of bed, put on a bathrobe and see your slender silhouette in the mirror. You put on fashionable clothes, a skirt and cute little blouse (or great trousers and shirt if you're a man) and leave for work. You feel great, especially after someone gives you a compliment. Later, you go for a walk, and there's a spring in your step with no extra weight to carry around. That night, you have fun planning what you'll be wearing to your next social event, knowing that you'll look fantastic.

Maybe it might be difficult for you to think about a person like that, because it seems so hard to imagine that such a person could exist. I'm here to tell you that they do, and you're going to discover them, and it's going to be wonderful. This book is all about how to find that slender person, the key ingredients and the knowledge that you'll need, and the work that you'll have to do to find them.

Before you read the rest of this book, you have an assignment to do.

Earlier, I asked you to think for a moment and imagine a slender you. Now, before you read the next chapter, you have a task to undertake. You need to create your own slender person and write down all your thoughts about them. That will be the first step that you take to help find the slender you. The task might only take an hour two. It doesn't really matter how long it takes, as long as you don't put it off forever.

Don't worry if you're not a good writer, because the only person who needs to read it will be you. But if you want to, you can talk about it with your friends or family. And you need to store the document you create because you're going to be using it again.

We all know that everyone is different, and every overweight person has a different history of weight gain. Some people were slim until after they had children, or gained weight as they grew older. Many others have been overweight all their lives or their weight has cycled up and down relentlessly.

If you've always been overweight, you'll need to think about your entire life as you create the slender you. But if you've only gained weight in the last few years, you don't need to think about your childhood at all. And if your weight keeps changing like the weather, then you'll need to begin with the time that started to happen.

What would your past have been like?

The first step in finding the slender you is to think about your past.

Why bother doing that? We all know that we can't change history, and the best approach is to correct problems today and then plan for a better future. There's no way that we can return to the past, before you had a weight problem, and change everything so that you never gain weight.

It would be great if we could travel back in time and change just that facet of our lives. I often thought to myself that I wished I hadn't gained that weight when I was pregnant, or gained weight again after losing it. I've even wished that I could wake up and find that I was slim, or lose weight quickly and easily. But I know that I was only dreaming.

There are two good reasons, though, why I want you to travel back in time, if only in your mind. The first reason is that thinking about your past will help you to remember when and why you gained weight. The second reason is that it will help to make that slender person more of a reality for you.

When writers create characters, they have to create a backstory for them. That's the term they use for the person's life before the real story starts. They need to think about what has happened to them in the past so that when you meet a character in a movie or book for the first time, they have a history and you're really halfway through their story without realising it. Look at Batman: Bruce Wayne was the son of wealthy philanthropists who were murdered by criminals. That happened in the past, but we meet him as an adult and we understand why he wants to be a crime fighter. Do you remember the Phantom? His family had been fighting crime for several generations, so he had a long backstory before we meet him for the first time in comic books.

You're going to create a backstory for the slender you because soon the real story is going to begin and you're going to be the star. Creating this story will definitely be the hardest thing that there is to do in this book. Once you've done that, everything else will seem very simple.

Now I want you to use your imagination and do some serious thinking. If you're searching for someone, you have no hope of finding them unless you know a little bit about them and their appearance. So sit down with a pen and paper, or at your computer, and start to describe them. It's very important to keep a written record, so that you can refer to it any time you want. You'll be amazed at what you find.

Just remember that this person is you – a slender you – so you're really describing yourself. They have the same head and heart as you, so they're not a stranger. They look out from behind your eyes, look downwards and see your body. Have you ever looked out from behind your eyes at that body you're attached to, and dreamed of looking down at a slender person? I know I have, so many times.

First of all, think about your past. Imagine if you'd always been slim. What would your childhood have been like? What would you have done? Would you have played more sport, looked great in your best clothes, felt more like the other kids?

If you weren't overweight as a child, you don't need to write about your childhood. Just begin your backstory whenever you started to gain weight.

As you grew older, what would you have done? Would things have been different if you were slim? Would you have had the courage to pursue more of your dreams, felt better about yourself, had more romances? Would you have had more fun as a teenager? Describe what life might have been like for the slender you.

This is only your imagination, so you can make up any story that you like, as long as it's something you would have wanted and might have dared to do if you'd been thinner. Perhaps your weight problem affected your career or life choices. Try not to go too far down that path, because the reality is where you are now.

You don't have to write a long story, and you can just write a few notes if you wish. Try not to dwell too much on negative or sad things that might have happened to you. Feel excited and happy as you create this character, because soon you'll have a very big adventure of your own.

Then imagine this slender person's life right up until the age you are now. Would it have been very different to yours? Remember that they would have the same family and friends as you, and the same thoughts and feelings.

I know how awful I felt as a primary school child when I went through a phase of being quite fat. My slender person would have been a slim child, who never felt different to the other kids. I was slim in sixth grade, but the other kids still remembered and I didn't get invited to dance with a boy at the all-important sixth grade dance. My slender child would have been able to wear all the latest fashions, not just outfits chosen with my difficult figure in mind, that awful girl in her class would not have bullied her, and she would have had at least one boy ask her for a dance.

During my thirties, when I should have been at my best, I dressed in ghastly clothes and thought constantly about losing weight. We were living on an Air Force base, and I didn't want to attend the annual ball because I knew that I felt so bad about my appearance. My slender person would have enjoyed that wonderful time, looked fantastic at all the social events and lived every day to the full.

What would you be like now?

You're halfway through creating that slender person, and your next task is a bit easier and probably more fun. You need to think about the slender you right now: the person you would be today if you were slim. Can you imagine that?

First of all, think about what you might be like today if you'd always been thin. Write down today's date and describe them. Talk about what they might be wearing, what they might look like, and what they might be doing. Would they be at home, or would they be at work? What would they do in their spare time? Would they go for a walk with friends and have coffee, or work out at a gym, or perhaps play golf or ride a bike? You can even take some photos from a magazine or the Internet that show what the slender you might look like or what they might be doing today.

Make sure that the slender you is doing things that you'd like to do. If you're a person who would never want to do extreme sports (like me), then don't write that the slender you will go mountain climbing or bungee jumping. You can mention jogging, even if you currently get exhausted after walking to your mailbox. But you need to keep grounded in reality. If you know that you have a disability and couldn't ever go jogging, or even walking, then don't write that down – unless you think that losing weight will improve your mobility. And thinking that the slim you might be a supermodel or Hollywood star could be going a bit too far: there's only a few people in the world like that!

I used to hate exercise, and never wanted to walk any distance. Maybe you've stopped exercising, and don't think it's something that you'd ever want to do. But I can assure you that the slender you will definitely like it. So at least write down some form of exercise that you know you'd be capable of doing if you were slim. Doesn't it make the slender you sound more interesting?

Perhaps the slender you (whether you're a man or a woman) is shopping for clothes today. They're going to walk around the stores trying on stylish clothes in smaller sizes that fit them perfectly and make them look fabulous. No one looks at them in a patronising way and tells them they don't stock their size. They walk right past the large-size shops. You could look at today's fashions and describe exactly what the slender you will buy or wear today.

If you have children or grandchildren, perhaps the slender you will take them to the park and have a wonderful time running around. They might even be the best looking Mum or Dad there.

You've finished the first step on your weight loss journey

Take plenty of time to finish writing about the slender you. Leave it for a day and come back to it: you might have some more ideas. I hope you found that interesting to think about, and that it made you wish that you could be a bit more like that person. Don't be upset though, because this is a time to be excited and happy. You're going to learn a wonderful secret soon because you're going to learn how to become that person.

So far, you've done very well. Thinking about the slender you is definitely the most difficult thing that you'll be asked to do in this book. After that, you'll find everything else is very straightforward.

If you believe that you can become the slender you, then you've taken the very first step on your weight loss journey. Belief is the first key ingredient to weight loss. Believe with all your heart that you can become that slender person. That will give you a goal, and help to keep you motivated.

Chapters 5 – 25 are about the second key ingredient to weight loss: knowledge. The One Way Diet is not just a healthy eating plan, but is also about coping with every aspect of your weight loss journey. That's why these chapters cover a wide range of topics.

CHAPTER 5: WHY WE GAIN WEIGHT SO EASILY

How our ancient past affects us

Have you ever seen those beautiful black cabs that drive around London and are such a prominent part of that historic city? The taxicab drivers need to pass a very difficult test to obtain a licence. They have to memorise all the major traffic routes in London, and it usually takes two or three years of study and at least ten attempts at the test before they finally manage to pass. The information that they need to master is called *The Knowledge.*

Now it's your turn to gather the knowledge you need so that you know how to lose weight. Luckily, though, you don't need to study for years and there are no tests. You just have to relax, put your feet up and read this book. You don't need to memorise it, because you can refer to it as often as you want. I'm not saying that this is the only place you can find that knowledge, but this book will give you a start.

Have you ever wondered why you gain weight so easily, and why your body stores fat so easily? It isn't just your fault or the fault of your parents. And it isn't just because you have a sweet tooth or eat too much each day.

They say that about sixty per cent of Australians, Americans and British people are overweight now, so you have plenty of company. Is being overweight a normal state? Why is weight gain spreading like an epidemic in our society? Is it a disease? To help you understand how to lose weight you need to understand why your body gains weight. And to do that, you need to think about the distant past when humans lived as nomadic hunters and gatherers.

Epidemics are infectious diseases caused by germs spreading from one person to another. Sometimes the germs spread indirectly via something else, such as the water supply or an insect. When a large number of people in a community catch an infectious disease we call it an epidemic and say that it's spreading quickly. Some well-known infectious diseases are the common cold, influenza, cholera, tuberculosis and malaria.

Obesity isn't an infectious disease, and it isn't a true epidemic. Weight gain is not a disease at all, but it can help many diseases to develop. If you are overweight you increase your chance of developing all sorts of diseases such as arthritis, heart problems, diabetes and even cancer. Being overweight puts a big strain on your muscles, bones and heart, just because of the extra weight load.

Try filling up your car boot with something heavy and driving it around. You can feel your car struggling and going slower, can't you? And try walking up a hill with two bags full of oranges slung over your shoulders. You'll be lucky if you don't get a strained muscle or two.

Weight gain is really just a natural process in the body. We were designed and built for a very different way of life, one that lasted for a hundred thousand years. In those ancient times, people who were skinny and struggled to gain any weight probably had trouble surviving. Many of them would have died when times were tough, leaving the well rounded to survive. So is it any wonder that there are so many people now who put on weight so easily?

Our modern societies have been developing for just a few thousand years. But for a hundred thousand years before that, humans lived as nomadic hunters and gatherers. At first, they didn't even have fire, or it was used for warmth in winter and protection from wild animals at night. There was no cordon bleu cooking in those days.

What did people eat in those ancient times? Let's picture them somewhere in Europe fifty thousand years ago. They wandered around, gathering everything edible that they could find. There would be fruit, nuts, berries, and some wild grains. At certain times of the year these would be plentiful, but in the colder months they would be hard to find. People would probably also eat a few insects and little edible creatures, but please don't try that now! Some of those can be extremely toxic to humans.

Occasionally, when people were feeling particularly brave and hungry, they would hunt for meat. That was not easy when all you had for a weapon was a homemade spear or club made of wood. They would also catch fish from the ocean or rivers and streams.

The closest thing to a sweet treat was honey. A volunteer would raid a wild beehive and get quite a few bee stings in the process. If it was that difficult to get a piece of candy today, I wonder how many of us would feed that sweet tooth of ours?

Have you ever seen a cat eating a mouse? The first thing it does, after killing the poor creature, is to bite off its head and then devour the internal organs, including the intestines loaded with half-digested food. People would probably have done the same thing when they caught an animal, which would give them a stomach full of mixed grains.

Perhaps you're thinking that our early days sound ever so slightly idyllic, wandering about in the countryside picking fruits and berries. But there would have been droughts and even fires, when the source of food was drastically reduced. And every year there was near starvation when the long, cold winter came with hardly any food available. How did our ancestors manage to survive?

The ability to gain weight was vital for people to get through those difficult months. Luckily, they could eat their fill in summer and gain plenty of weight. Then, when the bad times came, and they needed to keep warm and live off their own bodies, they had a nice store of fat. Their weight would increase dramatically and then drop dramatically every single year. Does that sound like a form of yo-yo dieting to you?

About ten thousand years ago, humans began to develop agriculture. They planted grains, fruit and vegetables, raised animals for a ready source of meat and milk, and improved their fishing methods. They traded and stored their food, and had access to food all year long. They had to work hard, though, and the food they ate was very rough and unprocessed, so there wasn't much chance for people to gain a great deal of weight.

One hundred years ago processed foods such as cake mixes, sauces, breakfast cereals, jams and frozen dinners were unavailable. Meals, cakes and treats had to be made from scratch. Many people did strenuous physical work every day, so they were able to eat a bit more without getting fat. Poor people would often struggle just to keep their family fed. For everyone, eating at a restaurant was a rare event and candy was only given to children on special occasions.

Today food has never been so readily available to so many people. All those processed foods, which are often high in fat and sugar, fill the supermarket shelves. Many people eat frequently at restaurants, cafes, all you can eat buffets and fast food restaurants. But our bodies have not evolved to cope with this out-of-control over-nutrition. Our bodies want to store all that extra food so that we can survive a few months of starvation. Is it any wonder that so many people are becoming overweight?

Hunger and why we need food

Have you ever wondered why we become hungry, or why we find eating so enjoyable? We love all the wonderful flavours and textures of food, and when we become hungry we try to find something to satisfy our appetite.

The truth is that those feelings of hunger and our pleasure in eating are really just instincts that Mother Nature has given us. They're essential because without them we would probably starve. All of our instincts have been given to us for the purpose of keeping us alive, and the instinct to eat is no different. The real reason for having instincts, as with any other animal, is to ensure survival of the species.

Imagine if you never felt hungry and never enjoyed the taste and sensation of eating, so that everything you chewed had no flavour at all. You would have no desire or motivation to eat, and wouldn't even think about it. You might completely forget to eat, or simply not bother to prepare any food. Gradually, your weight would drop so much that you might even die.

Today, we can observe that effect when people lose their sense of taste because of an accident or illness. Those people have to force themselves to eat, and desperately miss the pleasure they used to derive from eating. Have you ever been ill and lost your appetite, even for just a day or two?

You might think that would be wonderful for your diet, and wish you could stop the pangs of hunger or thoughts about eating whenever you looked at some food. But you need to remember that they are just instincts that are essential to your survival, and without them your life would be quite miserable. You should never blame yourself for that hunger, or tell yourself that you are greedy or gluttonous.

Why does your body need food? We need food because it provides us with nearly everything we need to keep us alive. It's essential to our survival. We can survive just a few days without water, and a few weeks without food.

What does your body do with the food you eat? You have a very complex digestive system designed to supply what your body needs to use and store the leftovers. Your body doesn't let anything go to waste and converts excess food into a store of fat. It makes the best use of your food so that you could survive all those periods of starvation that we endured in our ancient past.

Just imagine a factory that was able to make 100 cars every day. At the end of one day, the salesman says that 80 cars have been sold. So what does the factory manager do? Does he throw out the remaining 20 cars that they made? No, of course he doesn't! He keeps them in storage, hoping that someone will buy them tomorrow or the next day. The following day they sell 120 cars, so they really needed those extra cars in storage.

Now think about us. Each and every day we take in more food than we need so that our bodies have to put some of our food supplies into storage as fat. Gradually, over time, we keep building up storage supplies and much to our surprise our weight keeps increasing. Oh, dear. Unfortunately, we can't tell our bodies that they don't need to store our food as fat reserves any more.

What we can learn from our ancient past

So what can we learn from considering how humans lived in the ancient past? First of all, we need to eat a wide variety of foods because that is essential for good health. In the past, though, food was hard to obtain at certain times of the year.

We know that weight gain is just a natural process. You eat food, and then your body uses what it needs and stores the rest as fat.

Long ago those fat supplies would help to keep us alive during a famine. But now, we have access to plentiful food all the time. These days, we don't need those extra fat reserves.

Our hunger and the pleasure we derive from eating are really just instincts to make sure that we keep eating. That is essential for survival. Once again, our bodies don't realise that we don't need all those fat stores any more.

So here we are in the modern world, with all those hunger pangs and tendencies to gain weight. How can we find a way to control all those natural processes? The next chapter is about how our bodies make use of the food we eat.

CHAPTER 6: YOUR FRIENDLY DIGESTIVE SYSTEM

The food we eat

There are no special secrets, potions, supplements, treatments, magic foods or special inventions that can help you lose weight. Without realising it, you have eaten more than you needed and your body has stored that extra food as fat reserves. You didn't want it to, but your body thought you would need those reserves to help you survive a famine. Your job now is to get rid of that extra fat.

This is a very important chapter, because it contains some essential knowledge about what types of food you need and why each one important. You know that your body will use whatever food it needs and store the rest as fat. If you learn a little bit about how those fat reserves get created then you will have the knowledge to get some control over the situation.

Have you ever noticed that when you talk to a friend or colleague about a problem, or when you pray or meditate, you feel much better? You get a sense of control because talking or thinking about something helps you to understand it better and deal with your problems. It's the same when people are worried about some medical symptoms. When they get an accurate diagnosis from the doctor, they can feel much calmer and more in control.

That's why you need to learn a little bit about your digestive system and how your body uses food. If you are embarking on a long journey to find the slender you, you need to understand what you are doing. Just imagine the captain of a ship who didn't know anything about how a ship functioned. The ship would run aground before leaving the first harbour.

It is the same with your own body and that weight loss journey. You will become the captain of your own ship, know about your own body, and steer the course you want to discover the slender you.

Do you think that petrol is the most important thing you need to keep your car travelling along the road every day? It's the fuel that gives your car the energy it needs and if there is no petrol your car won't start. But your car also needs some other special things such as oil and water to keep it in great condition and occasionally it needs some repairs and a replacement part or two.

Imagine your car without petrol, without oil and water and with a few broken bits and pieces that you haven't had repaired or replaced. It's not going to go very far, is it? In fact, it is totally useless. You can try adding petrol but that won't help because you still need those repairs. Then you can try doing the repairs but you're still going to need oil and water as well.

That's what you would be like without food, because your body is a machine just like your car but infinitely more complex. Food supplies us with fuel energy, building blocks to do repairs and maintenance and special nutrients. All those things are essential to keep us alive and healthy.

There are just three major categories of food: proteins, carbohydrates and fats. That's it. They all do different things in the body, and we need all of them in our diet. What do you think is more important for your car: petrol, repairs and maintenance, or oil and water? The answer is that your car can't do without any of them, because they are all equally important. And your body is the same.

Think about what your body needs to do every day. It needs to operate all the parts of a very complicated machine that includes your heart, brain, lungs, bones, muscles and every other part of the body. When you walk, eat, talk, breathe or do anything at all, the cells of your body need energy. Some parts of the body such as our blood and skin are always being replaced, and other parts need running repairs. We also need to fight disease.

Even if we lay in bed all day, our bodies would still need to carry out all those activities. You might think you are resting, but your body is still hard at work. As you can imagine, your digestive system is very busy processing food for all those activities.

Proteins are just like the replacement parts for your car. When you eat protein foods such as meat, fish, eggs, nuts, dairy products and legumes, your intestinal system breaks them down into little pieces called amino acids. Those are the building blocks that you need to repair and replace things in your body.

Carbohydrates give you fuel energy and also supply some special nutrients. Carbohydrate foods are like the petrol you put in your car. You always put petrol in your car because you know how essential it is. So why would you decide not to eat carbohydrates?

Fat and oils, in extremely small amounts, are an essential part of your diet. You need to eat some fat to give you an extra energy source, help absorb fat-soluble vitamins and do some other important things like making cell membranes and hormones.

Everybody has some fat in their body, and a small amount is essential to act as a cushion and to help keep us warm. Our fat reserves are inside our abdomen and chest, around our vital organs, and all over our bodies underneath our skin.

Fat can be found associated with most protein products, especially meat and chicken. Vegetable oils are excellent sources of fat. The fats you don't want or need to eat are trans-fats, which are found in most high-fat processed foods. They can be harmful for your cholesterol levels, which will increase your risk of a heart attack.

Fuel for our body

Petrol is the fuel that keeps your car going until you reach your destination and find a parking spot. You never drive your car for twenty-fours a day, and when you park your car then it stops using petrol and stays completely at rest.

Your body is different, and really quite amazing. It works non-stop without a break until the day you die, which might be for ninety years or even more. Isn't it incredible how that complex machine keeps going? If you buy a toaster or another gadget these days, you are lucky if it lasts for five years. But all through every day of our lives our body keeps functioning and needs a source of fuel.

Imagine if the level of petrol dropped too low in your car. You'd have to top it up with some more fuel. And your body is exactly the same. To work at its best, it needs a steady supply of fuel.

Your digestive system breaks down carbohydrates into glucose, which is the special fuel that we use in our bodies. Glucose gives your body the quick energy in your blood stream that is needed for everything you do each day. As long as there is a steady, twenty-four-hour supply of glucose in your blood stream then your body has all the energy it needs.

But it isn't possible to eat carbohydrates all through the day so that you have a steady flow of glucose. That's why your body has a complex and extraordinary system to keep you supplied with just the right amount.

Your body converts carbohydrates to glucose. But it also has two reserve tanks of fuel that can be converted to glucose when the levels drop too low and more glucose is needed. The first reserve tank of fuel is glycogen, which is stored in your muscles and liver. That can be converted to glucose quickly and easily. The second reserve tank of fuel is your store of fat. That can be converted to glucose, but it takes more effort and is a more complicated process. So it's only used after your glycogen stores are used up.

Your body will start to use up your fat reserves if you don't eat enough fuel supplies for your body's daily needs. That is how your body fat starts to disappear!

There is also a reverse side to all of that. When you eat carbohydrates, they get quickly converted into glucose to give you fuel for your body. But if you eat too many carbohydrates, that glucose gets converted into glycogen and stored in your muscles and liver. When your glycogen storage tanks become full, some glycogen gets converted to fat for storage. Oh, dear! And when you eat too many proteins or fat, the body will use what it needs, and the rest will be converted to fat for storage. Oh dear, Oh, dear! That is how we gain weight!

The bad news is that any type of food can be converted to fat storage if you eat too much of it. The great news is that your fat reserves can be converted to glucose and used for fuel if you eat less than your body needs. And that's how you lose weight!

A special word about carbohydrates

Carbohydrates can be either sugars or starches. It's important to know the difference between these, so that you know why everyone tells you to eat complex carbohydrates and avoid simple carbohydrates (sugar products).

Simple carbohydrates contain sugar. Biscuits, cakes, lollies, jam, honey and sugary cereals all contain sugar. The bad news is that these products get broken down very quickly and easily, so they give you a sudden spike of glucose in your blood. That glucose is used up very quickly and then your glucose levels drop quickly.

If your only source of carbohydrate is sugar products, then your glucose levels will be up and down throughout the day like a yo-yo and you will feel hungry again shortly after eating. Those spikes in glucose levels are especially bad if you are at risk of getting diabetes.

Complex carbohydrates are starches and these are broken down slowly into glucose. They give you a steady supply of glucose energy throughout the day and stop you feeling hungry and tired. Wholemeal breads, high fibre cereals, rice and potatoes all contain starches. They also give you fibre, which is essential for your bowels, and some other good nutrients.

Fruit and vegetables are complex carbohydrates, and are incredibly important. They give you all sorts of wonderful, life-giving nutrients, vitamins and minerals. Scientists are always discovering the special value of different sorts of fruits and vegetables.

When glucose runs out, your body will quickly turn stored glycogen into glucose for energy. That way, it keeps a steady level of fuel in the blood stream all through the day. But if you eat too many carbohydrates, then your glycogen storage tanks gets full, your body can't store any more, and the rest is converted to fat. Those fat reserves will stay there until they are needed as your body's source of energy.

The exciting news for you is that the time has come to use up those excess fat reserves and you can say goodbye to them forever.

CHAPTER 7: YOUR METABOLISM

How much food do you need each day?

You know that your car needs petrol, but how much do you put in your car each week? I bet that you know the capacity of your car's petrol tank, and how much petrol will keep your car running for a week or two. When you fill up your vehicle, you're always careful to use the right type of fuel. You certainly don't try to add any strange concoction that shouldn't be there because you're aware that just a few contaminants can do a great deal of damage to the engine. And you don't keep pouring in petrol after your tank is full.

It's a shame that we don't always take the same care with our own bodies. Do we know how much food we really need? Carbohydrates, proteins and fats are all an essential part of our diet, but they can all be converted to fat reserves if we eat too much.

We know that our body uses carbohydrates, proteins and fats to provide us with everything we need. We also know that we need all of those food groups to keep us in fantastic working order. Now that most of us live a much longer life, the last thing we want is to harm ourselves by depriving our body of something it needs. We want to stay healthy and happy and even improve our health. But how much food do we need to keep our bodies healthy?

Proteins, fats and carbohydrates can all be converted into body fat if we eat too much. Our fat reserves can be converted into energy but only when they're needed. We want to make our bodies use up those fat reserves so that we'll lose weight in the best possible way! But we also need to make sure that we are able to manage our hunger, give our bodies what they need and stay healthy all at the same time.

It really is a balancing act. You need to find out how much food you need and it would be helpful if you could measure it, just like you can measure your height in centimetres or your weight in kilograms. Luckily, there's a very easy way to measure our food.

Food can be measured by the amount of energy it provides. Food energy is measured in *calories* or *kilojoules*. Kilojoules are the metric measurement, and calories are the pre-metric imperial standard. I like calories because I think they are much smaller, easier numbers to remember and to add up.

Have you heard the words *calorie* or *kilojoule* and wondered what they really meant? They're units of measurement, just like kilograms or centimetres or litres. They're terms that are very important for weight loss.

Every type of food item provides you with a different amount of energy. It's a complicated scientific process to work out the number of calories in a food item, but luckily we can leave that to the food technologists and scientists to calculate. Fortunately, there are wonderful food labels now that show the kilojoules or calories in any food we buy. And there are great websites or booklets where you can check the calorie content of any sort of food. There will also be estimates of the calories that might be in a cake or other recipe.

How many calories of food do you need each day? Women need about 2,000 calories (8,373 kilojoules) of food energy each day to maintain their current body weight, and men need about 2,400 calories. That is a very rough average, and depends on your age, size and activity levels. Unfortunately, as you get older, you tend to need fewer calories. There is no hard and fast rule, and everyone will require a different number of calories. People who lead sedentary lives will need fewer calories. Athletes who train for hours every day will need more.

If you eat less than that your body needs you will start to use up your fat reserves. There is no other way to get rid of them than to eat less than your body needs each day. That's all there is to it.

Now for two very special numbers: 1,200 and 1,500. If you are a woman you need to eat about 1,200 calories a day for steady, successful weight. If you are a man you can eat about 1,500 calories per day. You must avoid eating less than that and you shouldn't eat much more than that.

What would happen if you kept eating less than that? Wouldn't you lose more weight? The answer to that is an emphatic *no*. In fact, your weight loss will slow down or stop because your body will think it is starving and slow down your metabolism. That is how we managed to survive in ancient times when we were starving through those long, cold winters.

And there are all sorts of other nasty things that will happen to your body if you eat less than 1,200 calories a day (or 1,500 calories for a man). You'll feel tired and hungry. You'll develop thin bones and brittle nails. Your blood pressure and blood sugar levels will drop. You'll get an irregular heartbeat, your hair will fall out and your menstrual cycle will stop. And your body won't get all the nutrients and essential fuels that it needs. You'll also become so hungry that your brain will tell you to overeat.

Doesn't that all sound terrifying? So don't even think about trying to eat less than 1,200 calories. You can eat a bit more, though, and still lose weight. Your weight loss will just be bit slower.

In the next chapter you can learn about how much of the different types of food you need to make sure that you have a steady supply of glucose, some protein and a bit of fat in your diet. And there are also some ways to control your hunger.

How fast do you use your food?

How long does a full tank of petrol last? If you only drive once a week it might last for a month. But if you're on a long journey, it might only last a day. Fuel consumption is usually measured as the number of litres needed for a one hundred kilometre trip. If you are travelling on a highway, your car might have a fuel consumption rate of seven litres of petrol per one hundred kilometres. But in the inner city, your car might use twelve litres of fuel per one hundred kilometres. The rate of fuel consumption in your car is never constant, and increases when it has to work harder. Try driving up some steep hills and look at the fuel consumption rate on your dashboard monitor.

Our bodies are exactly the same. If we're very active, our bodies burn fuel at a faster rate. If we're slow and sitting down all day, our bodies need less fuel. And just like different makes and models of cars, each one of us has a different rate of burning fuel. We all need a different amount of fuel each day to maintain our current weight.

Our fuel consumption rate is called our *metabolism*. The rate we burn up calories in our body is our *metabolism* or *metabolic rate*. You don't need to understand it precisely, or measure your exact metabolic rate. All you need to do is understand the general concept.

The reason every person needs a different number of calories is because each person has a different metabolism. Each one of us is different, and some have a rapid metabolism. Do you know someone who seems to eat tons of food without gaining weight? They must have a fast metabolism. Some people have a slow metabolism, and put on weight easily. Plenty of exercise or physical activity will increase your metabolism and burn up more calories.

Our car's fuel consumption is very similar, although in that case we want the opposite outcome. We would love to have a fuel-efficient car that burns up a low amount of fuel per kilometre. We don't want a gas-guzzler that consumes fuel at a great rate. When it comes to ourselves, though, we'd love it if we could burn up heaps of calories each hour. That would really help us to lose weight, and would also mean we could eat everything in sight and still keep a trim figure.

How to keep your metabolism revved up all day

Your car will use up more fuel if it has to work harder and your body is exactly the same. If you keep your metabolism revved up all day you will use up the calories that you've eaten and then start to burn off your fat reserves. Your weight loss will be faster and you will feel healthier. And, as an extra bonus, you will feel energised instead of feeling slow and sluggish.

How can you keep your metabolism revved up all day? The first and most efficient method is to eat six times a day, starting with breakfast and finishing with an evening snack. As soon as you start to eat, your metabolism turns on the ignition switch and gets into gear. By eating throughout the day, your metabolism stays in high gear and keeps on burning those calories. If you skip breakfast and don't eat anything until lunchtime, your metabolism stays in ultra-slow mode all morning.

The second way to keep your metabolism at full speed is to be active and do some exercise. I'll talk much more about exercise in a later chapter. It isn't hard to believe that doing some exercise, even just a short walk, will increase your metabolism because it means your body has to do more work. The amazing thing is that the effect on your metabolism will last all day, not just while you're actually doing the exercise.

Try to think of some ways to be more active if you have a sedentary lifestyle. If you work at a desk all day, stand up and move around more frequently and go for a walk at lunchtime. Try to do more gardening or some household chores so that you are not sitting down all day. You'll feel much better and it will help your weight loss.

You know how much food you need, why you need it and how fast your body uses it. In the next chapter you'll learn all the practical aspects of designing a healthy 1,200-calorie eating plan (or 1,500-calorie plan for men).

Keep reading, and it won't be long before you're ready to start that journey to find the slender you.

CHAPTER 8: THE ONE WAY HEALTHY EATING PLAN

Why we need a healthy eating plan

Please remember that this is my personal healthy eating plan, and should not be regarded as professional advice about what you should eat. This is the diet I followed to lose weight, but you should see your physician or other qualified health professional before starting any weight loss program.

You know how your body seems to work against you in this modern world. You have easy access to food every single day, and you'd like to eat as much as you could with plenty of delicious food choices. You feel hungry, which is just a natural instinct to keep you alive. You don't want your body to store any extra fat reserves, because you don't really need them. But if you eat more than your body needs, the next thing you know is that you've gained some weight.

You know that to lose those fat reserves you need to eat at least 1,200 calories a day (or 1,500 calories for men) – but not much more than that. You also know that you need some carbohydrates, protein and fat in your diet. So why don't you just eat whatever you want, as long as some of those things are included, and stop when you get to the magic total of 1,200? Would you lose weight?

The answer is that yes, you would lose weight. But you would feel hungry for much of the day, and your body wouldn't get a well-balanced supply of energy and all the nutrients that it needs. You wouldn't feel healthy and happy, and you would soon stop your diet.

On a 1,200-calorie diet (or a 1,500-calorie diet for a man), you'd like to keep your metabolism revved up twenty-four hours a day so that your fat reserves get used quickly, you need a steady supply of energy to keep you alert and happy, and you need to get every single nutrient that your body needs. And you also need a good supply of fibre to keep your bowels working properly.

Doesn't that sound like the very best way to lose weight? But I'm afraid that doing it all by yourself is like walking a very precarious tightrope over a deep chasm. How much is too much? How many serves of the different sorts of food should you have? The only way to achieve success and become the slender you is to follow some ground rules for a healthy diet.

Most governments publish dietary or nutritional guidelines for different age groups. You can easily find these on the Internet, or ask your local library to help you. Those recommendations are based on sound scientific evidence, and they usually suggest a diet containing all the major food groups. Please don't listen to anyone who tries to tell you that you should cut anything out unless your doctor recommends this for an important, diagnosed medical reason.

If you follow all the grounds rules for a healthy diet then instead of taking each step slowly on that precarious tightrope, you'll walk quickly and confidently to the other side. You'll impress your friends and family and, more importantly, you will amaze yourself.

The Specifications for the One Way Diet

Have you ever heard of specifications? Just imagine that you want a kitchen makeover. A kitchen designer will draw a plan, but before they do that you need to have some specifications. They're all the things that you would like to have in your new kitchen. Your list might include a wall oven, lots of bench space, plenty of deep drawers, a space for a microwave oven and a stovetop. The designer will then draw a plan that includes all of those items.

There are some simple specifications for your healthy eating plan. If you're going to make it successfully to the end of your weight loss journey, your diet needs to meet a few basic requirements. Think about each one of them carefully.

Firstly, you need to eat fewer calories than your bodies need each day, so that it will use up your fat reserves. But you need at least 1,200 calories a day (or 1,500 calories for a man). If you eat less than that, your body will think you're starving and you also won't be able to supply your body with the good things it needs.

Secondly, you need to maintain a steady supply of fuel throughout the day so that your energy levels remain steady and you don't feel tired and hungry. You should eat six times throughout the day so that your body never thinks that it is starving. It won't slow down the rate of energy use and you won't feel too hungry.

Thirdly, you need the correct level of all the recommended food groups to maintain your health. You want a sensible and delicious eating plan, and this needs to include some water or other liquids.

Do you agree with all those specifications? Do you think they sound like something you could live with? Now read the rules for a healthy diet. See if you think that it meets all of those specifications.

Rules for a healthy eating plan – The One Way Diet

I must emphasise, once again, that this is the method I used, but before you attempt to follow this plan you should see your doctor and follow their advice.

Here are the simple rules to follow so that you can use the laws of nature to your advantage and slowly use up your fat reserves. They're easy rules to follow, especially with a little bit of practice.

Are you the sort of person who tends to have similar food each day, or are you the sort of person who likes something different all the time? Do you tend to plan your meals far in advance, or do you make your decisions right at the last minute? I must admit that I tend to plan meals in advance and like to eat a similar breakfast and lunch every day. The rules for a healthy diet can be followed by anyone, but you will need extra determination and a bit of extra thought if you like making decisions at the last minute. You need to make sure that you have everything you need in your kitchen cupboard, and then your plan will be very easy to follow. Mark this page in your book and always keep it handy.

Remember, these are my rules but you should seek the advice of your physician to plan your own healthy eating program.

The Rules

RULE 1

Keep a food diary to help you record the number of calories you eat. Measure your food portions, and calculate the number of calories in each item. Add it all up to get your daily intake of food.

RULE 2

Aim to eat 1,200 calories a day (or 1,500 calories for men). Definitely don't eat less than 1,200 calories a day, even for a short period of time.

RULE 3

Drink some water or other calorie free liquids each day. Black tea of coffee with no sugar (with some skim milk added if desired), diet soft drinks (sodas), soda water, and clear soups all count as liquids. It is not essential to drink 2 litres of water a day, and many people have medical conditions that mean they should not drink too much water. Never drink normal juices or soft drinks (sodas) because they're all full of sugar.

RULE 4

Eat six times a day. That means breakfast, a mid-morning snack, lunch, an afternoon snack, dinner and an evening snack. That will help to keep hunger away and your body won't think it's starving and then slow down your metabolism.

RULE 5

Eat small portions. It might be difficult getting used to those small portions, but soon you'll wonder what you were thinking when you piled your plate high. Be proud of yourself.

RULE 6

Remember it is not the end of your diet if you have a treat. You need to include some treats and if you have an "undiet day" then simply resume your diet the next day.

RULE 7

Now for the details about the food, and what you should include each day. Enjoy a wide variety of nutritious foods. Be creative in mixing up and trying new things, especially new fruits and vegetables.

RULE 8

Eat four serves (or six serves for a man) of complex carbohydrates. That means foods such as bread, cereal, pasta, noodles, potatoes and sweet potatoes. A serve is one slice of bread, half a cup of muesli, 1 cup of cooked porridge, 1 bread roll, 1 cup of cooked rice or 1 cup of low-calorie noodles.

RULE 9

Eat five serves of vegetables and two serves of fruit each day. A serve is one average piece of fruit or half a cup of cooked vegetables.

RULE 10

Eat two serves of no-fat dairy foods each day. A serve is one cup of skim milk (which might be for your tea or coffee each day), a small carton of no-fat flavoured yoghurt or a slice of fat-reduced cheese.

RULE 11

Eat one small serve of lean meat, fish, poultry, nuts or legumes each day. A serve consists of two eggs, 100 grams of cooked meat, chicken or fish, or one third of a cup of lentils or a very small serve of nuts. Be wary of nuts, as they are very calorie-dense.

RULE 12

You can add one or two mini-serves of protein such as one tablespoon of peanut butter or a small, slender slice of lean meat. This will give you a very small protein serve at breakfast or lunch.

RULE 13

You can add one extra food item as a treat. That could be a glass of alcohol, two sweet biscuits, or other snack foods that are less than one hundred calories.

RULE 14

Don't put butter or margarine on your bread, don't add sugar to your tea or coffee, don't fry foods, don't use rich sauces, and don't add mayonnaise or salad dressings. You won't miss any of those things, and they are secret, hidden calories. Use only a smear of spray oil when you're cooking, and learn to cook the low-fat way.

So there you have it. They're the rules I wrote for my own healthy eating plan. Do you think that they meet the specifications for a healthy diet? Now it's up to you to plan your menus, prepare your own food, cook the low fat way, and carefully add up your own calories. In another chapter I talk about cooking and give you some very simple recipes. I also talk about calorie-free foods, which are a wonderful invention!

A suggested meal plan that I followed

I know how difficult it is to be given a list of rules and then have to work out some meal plans without any help. To help get you started, I'm going to give you my typical daily meal plan. On my weight loss journey I ate six times a day and enjoyed every mouthful. In a later chapter there are more suggested options for each meal.

Daily Meal Plan

1.5 cups of skim milk – used in tea or coffee throughout the day

Breakfast

One slice of wholemeal toast

One tablespoon of peanut butter

Morning Snack

One medium pear

Lunch

Two slices of rye bread with a smear of mustard

One 40-gram slice of lean ham

Lettuce, tomato and cucumber

Afternoon snack

One medium apple

Dinner

100 grams of lean beef flavoured with herbs

Steamed pumpkin, carrot, zucchini, tomato and capsicum

100 grams of potato

Dessert: large serve of diet jelly

Evening Snack

Small tub of diet no fat flavoured yoghurt

Two light (reduced fat) sweet biscuits

GRAND TOTAL = 1,200 calories per day

That's it. Do you think you could cope with a meal plan like that? I was surprised how well I coped, and there is one thing I know for sure. There is nothing that tastes as good as the feeling of losing weight.

CHAPTER 9: MINI-GOALS

It will take time to reach your goal

You're ready to go. You can't wait to get started and race till you get to the finish line and meet the slender you. Then your life will be transformed forever and you'll hardly be able to stop smiling.

But wait a minute. Where is that finish line? And is it so far in the distance that you can hardly see it? You might have seen those weight loss advertisements promising that you could lose ten kilograms in five weeks or six kilograms in two weeks. If only that could be true, then it would take us just a few weeks to lose those fat reserves. No wonder we get attracted by promises like that.

But we all know that it's very difficult to lose more than half a kilogram per week or one kilogram at the absolute maximum. If you go on a very extreme diet, then you might lose a little bit more for a short period of time. If you want to lose weight and stay healthy at the same time, you should count on losing no more than half a kilo a week.

How much weight should you try to lose? First, carefully measure your height. Then find out the healthy weight range for your height. You can easily find those recommendations on the Internet or ask your doctor or pharmacist. My height is 166 centimetres, so my healthy weight range is 55-69 kilograms. Choose the upper limit, and aim for that.

That is all there is to it. When you reach that weight, you will find the slender you. Just imagine what you might look like. That is your final goal, so make sure you write it down somewhere. It's a very important number.

Now weigh yourself today. Do you have a good pair of bathroom scales at home, or can you get access to some on a regular basis? The most important thing is to be consistent. Naked and first thing in the morning would be ideal, but if not then weigh yourself in the same type of clothing, without shoes, at the same time of day. And always put your scales in the same place on a sturdy, flat floor. That will all help to ensure a consistent measurement.

So how did you go with that first weight measurement? Was it the first time you dared to weigh yourself for a while? It's a very difficult thing to do, but you'll be glad that you did. Now write it down. You'll be amazed in a few weeks because those scales will be telling you a different story, and looking back at your first measurement will make you feel very happy.

Now for some very simple mathematics. First, work out how many kilos you need to lose to get to your goal weight. Write it down, and then double that number. If you lose about half a kilo per week that is how many weeks it might take you to reach your goal. I had 27 kilos to lose. Doubling 27 kilos came to 54. So I expected my weight loss journey to take 54 weeks. That might seem like a long time, but remember that your body took even longer to build up those fat reserves, and now it needs a long time to reverse that process.

After reaching 65 kilos, I then went even further and lost several more kilos.

How much time will you take to reach your goal? That is your finishing line, but the race is long and slow, and can be frustrating. How can you endure such a lengthy journey?

Why you need mini-goals

Have you ever watched an Olympic marathon? The athletes run for forty-two kilometres, which is an incredible achievement. All the competitors start enthusiastically, but it isn't long before a few people drop out of the race. Then, as time goes on, the field spreads out and more athletes drop out, injured or exhausted. When the winner finally enters the arena, there is a huge cheer from the crowd. It is always a wonderful moment when the victor reaches the finish line.

Your weight loss journey is exactly like that. You are determined to reach that finish line and you know that your friends and family will be cheering you on right to the end. But how can you keep going every single day?

The solution is to have mini-goals. You need to take little steps and celebrate your achievements all the way to the end. Your first mini-goal can be to lose five kilograms. How much will you weigh then? Write it down, and then write down the five-kilo increments all the way to your goal weight.

Now look at your first mini-goal. You are going to lose five kilograms. Think about that and focus on it. Does that seem achievable? When you reach that weight you will feel very proud, and you should notice the difference. Give a cheer and celebrate! Tell yourself that you are incredible! Don't worry about all the months that it might take to reach your ultimate destination.

When you have achieved your first mini-goal, you will be keen to reach your second one. In fact, each time you reach a mini-goal you will be keener to reach the next one. You will feel yourself getting slimmer, you will look better, and you will fit into clothes that had become too tight. Wonderful!

Have you ever tried the sport of orienteering, or heard about it? Enthusiasts follow a set course in the countryside with various checkpoints, using a map and compass to help them. They know that eventually they will reach the finish line, but they always need to focus on finding each checkpoint. They can't think about that ultimate goal.

When you have mini-goals your weight loss journey will feel like an orienteering course instead of a marathon. You will follow your plan, mark-off each mini-goal as you come to it and celebrate your achievements. Then you can turn your thoughts to meeting the next checkpoint, and then the next one. Bit by bit you will reach the finish line and find the slender you.

Your choice of mini-goals is entirely your decision. It doesn't have to be a loss of five kilograms. You might choose smaller increments. There are all sorts of ways to measure your weight loss, and you can think about what measures you would like to use.

Weights and measures – how to measure your weight loss

On the first day of my weight loss journey I stood naked on the scales at 6 am (apologies for that horrible image) and recorded my weight. When I arrived home from work that afternoon, I stood on the scales again and was stunned to see that my weight had risen by two kilograms! How could that be? For the next few days I stood on the scales several times a day, and found consistently that my weight could increase by two kilograms throughout the day.

Then I started to weigh myself each morning, while sticking religiously to my healthy eating plan. Sometimes my weight stayed the same, and sometimes it even increased. What was happening? Had my diet failed in some way before it had barely started?

My friend at work told me that I was, "messing with my head." It turns out that weight can vary by about two kilos each day, increasing as the day progresses because of fluid levels in the body and the food we eat. And our weight can vary each morning because of variations in our fluid retention. Weight loss is not a steady, daily decline. It can often jump down quite suddenly, after staying steady or rising slightly for several days.

The very best approach is to weigh yourself once a week at a standard time and place. Ideally, that would be first thing in the morning. Use the same set of scales and keep them in the same location on a sturdy, level floor. Different scales can vary by kilograms, so don't compare your weight on another set of scales. Consistency is the key.

The scales won't tell you everything, though. You can choose to take your body measurements and keep a record of them. Your chest, waist and hips are a simple measure, and you can also measure your arms and thighs. Make sure that you take your measurements in the same spot on your body, though!

And there are some other fun ways to record your weight loss. Do you have a wardrobe full of clothes in different sizes? Sort through all your clothes and try them on. Find ones that you can almost fit into and put them aside. Try them on when you reach your next mini-goal. I hope you get a nice surprise and increase your clothing options at the same time. Then find some more that you might fit into after you lose a few more kilos.

Your body measurements and those clothes you're aiming to wear very soon can also be added to your mini-goals. And if you can think of anything else, then add that as well. Perhaps if you lost five kilos you would be able to put on that swimming costume of yours and use the local pool. Perhaps there is a social event or holiday in the near future that you are looking forward to. You would love to lose a few kilograms so that you look and feel better, and you have enough time. Add all those items to your list of mini-goals.

I found that a loss of about six kilograms would be roughly equal to a change of dress size. That meant I might drop from a size eighteen to a size sixteen. So you might like to use six kilograms as your standard mini-goal and see if you can fit into a smaller clothing size. Don't get discouraged though, because we all know how clothing sizes can vary so much from brand to brand, especially for women.

You don't have to measure your weight in kilograms. You might prefer to use pounds or stones. When I was a child, before we changed to the metric system in Australia, people recorded their weight in stones. There are fourteen pounds in a stone, and one stone equals 6.4 kilograms. If you lose 3.2 kilos that means you've lost half a stone, and that is quite a significant weight loss. So you have a right to feel very proud!

You might decide that you would like to record your weight using all of those units of measurements. You can easily find quick conversion tools on the Internet to help you. Just remember, though, that the golden rule is to weigh or measure yourself no more than once a week.

How to celebrate your mini-goals

Write a list of you mini-goals, focus on them, plan for them and look forward to them. When you reach each mini-goal give yourself a hug and a pat on the back, tell anyone who will listen, and celebrate. Achieving a mini-goal can give you so much pleasure it can be enough of a celebration all by itself. It's like winning an Olympic gold medal: nothing else is really needed to give you a great sense of satisfaction. But you should also take the time to have a celebration, because you deserve it and it will help you live life to the full.

How can you celebrate? Once upon a time if I felt I deserved a reward my first thought would be something associated with food. My favourite treats would be a meal at a restaurant, coffee and cake at my favourite café, or some chocolates.

How can you choose to celebrate reaching a mini-goal in a way that doesn't make you gain weight? You could enjoy coffee with a treat or dine at a restaurant provided that you choose healthy options that comply with your healthy eating plan. I'll talk about the challenges of eating out in a later chapter.

You can be creative, though, and think about dozens of way to celebrate that don't involve food. You could go for a walk in a beautiful park and then enjoy some coffee. You could buy a book or magazine, see a movie, watch your favourite old TV series all the way through, have some wonderful private time all to yourself, enjoy a beauty treatment or get a new hairstyle. You could go to the beach for a stroll, spend some time with someone special, go for a bike ride, listen to some music, have a bubble bath or start to plan that vacation. You could also visit an art gallery or museum, or a village filled with gift shops.

Perhaps you could go to your local department store and talk about a new way to do your make-up, or get some style advice in the fashion department. You could buy a piece of costume jewellery, some make up or a new handbag. You could have a wonderful afternoon browsing through some vintage stores to see what you can find. Try on as much as you can to see what fits you.

Just remember to celebrate and record your success each time you reach a mini-goal and your final destination won't seem so far away.

CHAPTER 10: THE MEANING OF MOTIVATION

The meaning of motivation

I know that I said there would be no magic formulas in this book and no wondrous new revolutionary way to lose weight. But there is one magic pill that you need each day to keep you travelling on your weight loss journey. That magic pill is motivation.

Believe that you will become the slender you. That is your ultimate goal. Think about it, look forward to it and plan what you will do when you get there. Then you will find the motivation that you need.

That motivation will make you take action to achieve your goal.

I've already mentioned that I love to travel on cruises. But every single day on those cruises I take a tablet to prevent seasickness. I'm very prone to motion sickness, and if I didn't take that medication, then I would develop nausea and a host of other symptoms. I probably wouldn't want to finish my journey, and I certainly wouldn't enjoy it.

Motivation has the same role to play on your weight loss journey. You won't become ill without it, but you definitely won't complete that journey. Every single day, you need to find a new dose of motivation so that you take the necessary action to achieve your goal.

What is motivation? How can you define it? Motivation is the special thought process in our mind that makes us take action to achieve a goal. It's the reason that we take action.

Think about a great swimmer who wants to win an Olympic gold medal. That is her goal, and she is highly motivated by such an exciting dream. So every day she finds the motivation that makes her take action. What does she do? She swims up and down the pool for hours and tries as hard as she can to win every swimming competition.

Then think about the everyday things in your life that you are motivated to do. What actions do you take and why? You may go to work because you are motivated to earn money and get satisfaction from doing a great job. You love your children and want to give them the best possible life, so you are motivated to take action each day to look after them very well. You want to have an enjoyable dinner, so you are motivated to take the action needed to prepare it. You're keen to have that new quilt, so you are motivated to work on your latest quilting project each night. You work on restoring that old car in the garage, so that one day you will be able drive it around. Everyone is motivated to do something.

Perhaps you didn't realise that when you do all those everyday things, you have set yourself goals and then motivate yourself to take action to achieve them. When I run out of milk, I'm highly motivated to go to the local store so that I can enjoy my next cup of coffee. When you want to watch your favourite TV show, you're highly motivated to turn on the television.

In order to take action, you need to have a goal. But what is the goal that you want to achieve? Your big goal is to become the slender you. That is why you need the key ingredient of belief. You need to believe with all your heart that you will become the slender you. You also have mini-goals, and you know how important they are. But your big goal will always be to become the slender you. Isn't that a wonderful thing to look forward to? What an exciting goal!

Another important goal can be an upcoming event in your life, perhaps twelve months in the future. You know that there is time to lose weight before you go on that vacation or wedding or big family gathering - and you will look wonderful. Losing weight might have a dramatic beneficial effect on your health problem, and that is one of the best goals of all. Just imagine what your doctor will say!

In the moment of clarity, you find the motivation to take action and lose weight. You are ready to go, like a racehorse in the starting gate waiting to run the Melbourne Cup. You are determined to get to the finish line, no matter what it takes. You have burned all the bridges behind you and there is no way to turn back. You are determined to lose all of your excess weight. You have the inspiration and you are determined to expend the necessary perspiration. Motivation is the magic pill that you need every day so that you take action to achieve your goal of becoming the slender you.

How to maintain your motivation

None of us do anything without motivation, so we need to think about it every single day. There are all sorts of wonderful, practical ways to increase your motivation and keep yourself motivated. You will then be inspired to achieve your goals. Your major goal will be to become the slender you and you will also have mini-goals along the way. Every time that you reach a mini-goal you will have an energising feeling of satisfaction and accomplishment.

If you are looking forward to a major event in the future, focus on that and use it as your major goal. Think about how wonderful you will look. Plan an imaginary wardrobe for yourself and look forward to wearing those wonderful clothes. And make sure there truly is plenty of time for you to lose that weight. You shouldn't expect to lose more than half a kilo each week, and you won't always lose that much.

You can go through your wardrobe and find some nice clothes that don't fit you anymore. Choose clothes that are a just a bit tight, and others that a size or two smaller. Try them on occasionally and see what you can fit into. When something fits you again, you'll feel very happy. Re-organise your closet and find some great clothes that you can't wait to wear again. I'll be talking more about clothes in a later chapter.

Take some photos of yourself before you start and take regular photos as you lose weight. How inspiring! Look at them regularly. And if you have a photograph of yourself when you were slim, then make a copy and keep it handy so that you can look at it all the time.

When people give you a compliment or make a remark that you look a bit thinner, write it down in a little book or a document on your computer. Refer to it on a regular basis. Cut out or download photos of fashion you want to wear or people you want to look like. Gather some more photos of yourself when you were thinner. Keep them somewhere safe and look at them frequently. You'll soon look like that again!

Do fun things that don't involve eating, like going for a walk somewhere beautiful, meeting a friend for coffee, seeing a movie, visiting another town or exploring a museum. All those activities will make you feel better. I'll talk more about exercising in another chapter. Take up a new hobby or learn a new skill. Write down a list of things that you might be interested in and select one of them to try.

Choose a movie or television hero or heroine that inspires you. One day, when you're slimmer, you'll look a little bit like them.

Feeling hungry or longing for a favourite treat is the biggest challenge you face, and it can ruin your motivation. If you have three snacks a day, though, as well as three meals, then you can space out your eating and help to keep hunger at bay. You can also have water, tea, coffee, diet soft drinks (sodas) and a variety of no-calorie or very low-calorie snacks. The occasional treat can also be very beneficial for a number of reasons. It can be thoroughly enjoyable, and it can have the added effect of kick-starting your weight loss if it has stalled briefly. We all need the occasional treat.

Sometimes, if you are really struggling, it's better just to get out of the house and go for a walk or go to bed and have a sleep. Your friends and family and other people in a weight loss club or online forum can be helpful and sympathetic. Talk to them as much as possible if you find that helps you. A diet buddy can be your best inspiration.

How to maximize your motivation every single day

You've thought about the importance of motivation and established some inspiring goals to give you that motivation. Now is the time to write them all down, gather any photographs that you need and keep a special folder full of everything that motivates you. It doesn't matter how often you look at it, as long as you look at it frequently and think about it even more.

It's important, though, that you also think about maximising your motivation every day. Each day is different and some days will be harder than others. There will be times when you're tired or upset about something, or sick of sticking to your weight loss program. That's when you'll need to maximise your motivation.

Just imagine trying to sew a dress with barely enough fabric to do the job. You try as hard as you can and stretch the fabric as much as possible. But when the job is finished, you can barely squeeze your body into it. Imagine instead if you had just a bit more fabric to work with. When the dress is finished you can slip it on easily, and it feels loose and comfortable.

That is the difference it makes when you maximise your motivation. It makes your struggles a little bit easier and helps you to cope very well each day. And it may mean the difference between success and failure on those difficult days.

How can you maximise your motivation? Look at your special list of goals and examine each one individually. Then think about how you can expand that goal, just a little bit, so that your motivation is increased for at least one day.

Have some extra calorie-free snacks if you are really struggling one day. And instead of thinking about fitting into that old blouse of yours, cut out the picture of a stunning jacket that you never thought you'd be able to wear. If your goal is to look very nice at that family wedding next year, think instead about looking totally stunning. Forget about your natural modesty and inhibitions.

You won't always need the same amount of motivation. When your weight loss program becomes routine, you'll only need a small dose of motivation each day. Often, you won't even think about it. But sometimes you will need a big dose and occasionally a huge dose. Unlike medication, there is no limitation to how much you should have. Take as much as you need every single day to help you along your journey.

Remember that you need to believe you will become the slender you. That is your goal and your motivation, the magic pill that will make you take action each day to achieve your dream.

CHAPTER 11: COOKING THE WEIGHT LOSS WAY

Some replacement therapy

You don't have to look very far to find some rich and delicious food to tempt you. Just open a cookbook, visit a friend or stroll along the street past cake shops, cafes and restaurants. Write down a list of your favourite dishes and see what they contain. Are there rich creamy sauces, cakes, biscuits or desserts loaded with butter, sugar, chocolate and cream, or deep fried foods covered in batter? Or how about a sandwich or salad with heavy lashings of mayonnaise?

Try looking up the calorie content of just some of your favourites. You might get a surprise to find that some of them would use up a large proportion of your daily calorie allowance. So while you might enjoy them for a few minutes, you could be hungry for the rest of the day and that would not be much fun.

I'm definitely not saying that you should never have your favourite foods again. You should regard those very rich foods as a great treat to indulge in occasionally. Life without those special treats would be very dull indeed and if you find yourself longing for something, then you should have a small serving and enjoy it.

The best way to survive a long weight loss journey is to eat as much delicious wholesome food as you can each day. That's why you need to learn some simple tricks for weight loss cooking. It's all about saving invisible calories, the sort that slip down your throat without you noticing.

Just imagine a ham and salad sandwich with lashings of mayonnaise on two slices of buttered bread. That will contain 420 calories. If you remove the butter or mayonnaise it will be 220 calories. A cup of full cream milk has 170 calories and a cup of skim milk has 85 calories. See what a difference it makes?

If you are going to travel on your weight loss journey for a long period of time, then you need to save as many calories as you can by learning to cook and prepare food the weight loss way. With a just a little bit of practice, you won't even notice that all those things you used to add to your food are missing, you will improve your health and you won't feel hungry.

The first thing to learn about is some replacement therapy. Then we'll talk about cooking the weight loss way and look at some simple recipes.

You might have heard about replacement therapy for a number of medical conditions. Luckily, the sort of replacement therapy in this book doesn't require a doctor's prescription, it will probably save you money, and won't be painful at all. In fact, it will make you feel great because you'll be able to eat more food each day.

You're going to replace some of the foods you eat now with more sensible choices. It will be great for your waistline, great for your hip pocket, and once you start a new way of thinking you won't even notice that those old foods are missing. You will love your new way of eating!

So what foods do you need to replace? Let's start with full cream milk. If you can replace it with skim milk you will save quite a few calories throughout the day. Skim milk is normal, natural, healthy milk that has simply had the fat removed. The fat content is also known as cream. All the other good things, such as protein and calcium, still remain.

And that brings me to the subject of tea and coffee. It's very fortunate that tea and coffee have zero calories, so they are a wonderful drink for people losing weight. But you need to stop adding sugar, and replace all the milk you add with just a small amount of skim milk. You can have those milky coffees as an occasional treat, but normally you should try to drink tea and coffee with no sugar and with either no milk or just a dash of skim milk.

When I was a child I was always given a cup of tea with heaps of full cream milk and two teaspoons of sugar. When I was a teenager I started to replace that creamy milk with the skim variety and over a week or two reduced the amount of sugar to zero. And do you know what happened? Ever since the, I've loved the light, refreshing taste of a cup of tea or coffee with no sugar and only a dash of skim milk. I loathe the taste of tea or coffee with creamy milk and even a minute amount of sugar. It will only take a few weeks to adjust, but you will also learn to love it.

You need to replace sugary soft drinks (sodas) with diet soft drinks (sodas) that have almost zero calories. After a while, you'll hate the cloying sweet taste of a normal soft drink. Did you know that a glass of soft drink (soda) could have about seven teaspoons of sugar dissolved in it? Fruit juices and cordials are also high in calories because of the sugar content. Try to replace them with a zero or almost-zero calorie drink. Instead of a fruit juice, replace that with a piece of fruit.

Try to cut back on adding sugar and salt to many of your foods. Salt does not have any calories, but can increase your blood pressure. Sugar can add many hidden calories when you add it to different items throughout a single day.

Butter and margarine are fat products that are dense in calories. When you make a sandwich or a piece of toast, don't use any butter or margarine. Once you add some spread or a slice of meat with plenty of salad, you won't even notice that the butter or margarine are missing. And you'll be saving heaps of calories.

Fat, oils, butter and margarine used for cooking should be kept to an absolute minimum. Recipes that use more than a dash of cooking oil will add many calories to the final product. Look at the product labels on any foods that you buy. If you see more than a minute amount of fat you'll also notice that the calorie or kilojoule content is very high.

You'll need to replace creamy sauces with low-calorie alternatives. I'll talk about cooking the weight loss way soon, and you'll find that there are all sorts of wonderful ways to make your food delicious, easy to prepare, and totally satisfying.

Sugary cereals are low in fibre and don't give you a long, slow, steady supply of glucose. You'll need to replace them with a cereal made from whole grains. You'll soon enjoy that sort of cereal much more, especially when you know how satisfied it makes you feel. If you also eat white bread or rolls you need to replace those with wholemeal varieties that will give you energy for so much longer.

Mayonnaise and other high fat dressings need to be replaced with low fat varieties or avoided altogether. Don't eat ice cream, dessert sauces and full cream yoghurts. If you search your supermarket shelves you will find some low calorie tubs of dessert or yoghurt. Check the labels carefully to see the calorie content, and try them.

Cream, as most of you will agree, is delicious and I love to add it to a rich dessert on a special occasion. But you need to avoid it while travelling on your weight loss journey, or just have one tablespoon of the whipped variety as an occasional treat.

Chocolates, candy, candy bars and chips should be avoided if possible, or used as a very rare treat. If you check the calorie count of your favourites, you will soon see why.

Takeaway foods and other high fat foods need to be replaced with healthy, low calorie alternatives. Sometimes, especially when travelling, they can be hard to avoid but they definitely won't help your weight loss journey.

Methods for weight-loss cooking

Now the time has come to learn a new way to cook. But there is no need to despair, as learning to cook the weight loss way is very easy and inexpensive. It will only cost you a few dollars at your local supermarket and you'll be an expert in no time.

First, you need a can of cooking spray oil. Any sort will do, but if possible try to use olive oil because it has all sorts of health benefits. You also need a small container of olive oil or other vegetable oil. That's it. Did you know that spray oil has almost no calories so it is just great to use for cooking? It sprays cooking oil droplets in such a thin layer that it barely amounts to any oil and yet is a great medium for cooking food.

Now look for some basic ingredients in your pantry cupboard. On the spice racks try to find some garlic, chives, pepper, stock cubes, potato sprinkles and any other herbs that you like. They have virtually zero or very low calories. Buy some cans of tomato, some oyster sauce and some packs of diet jelly. That is enough to get you started.

Now for two simple lessons. First of all, let's try one fried egg on toast. Heat your favourite frypan and spray lightly with cooking spray. Break one egg into the centre of the frypan, heat until cooked and place on one unbuttered slice of wholemeal toast. That's it! You've started to cook the weight loss way.

Now for lesson two. Peel a 150 g piece of potato or sweet potato. Cut into slices or wedges, spray with cooking spray and dust with potato sprinkles and pepper. Place on a baking tray that has been lightly greased with cooking spray. Now bake for about fifty minutes on medium heat. You're already an expert and you'll enjoy eating what you've created.

A few simple recipes

I would never claim to be a great chef who spends half their day in the kitchen creating exotic recipes. You won't see me trying to be a celebrity chef, and I don't have any dreams about opening my own restaurant or writing a cookery book. It's very fortunate for me that cooking the weight loss way is so simple.

Here are a few of my favourite dishes to help get you started. After that, you'll be able to create your own delicious recipes. Some of them can be frozen so they can be quickly reheated for an easy healthy meal when you arrive home after a busy day.

Spicy Vegetable Medley

Ingredients: Choose a wide variety of vegetables that are suitable for baking. Some of these include: pumpkin, capsicum, cherry tomatoes (cut in half), zucchini, celery, potato, sweet potato, parsnip, carrots, onion, turnip, beetroot, cucumber, yellow squash and spring onions. A serving for one person is about 180 grams in total.

Wash, peel and chop the vegetables into chunks. Combine in a bowl with 2 tablespoons olive oil, 2 tablespoons of minced garlic and 2 tablespoons of finely chopped chives. Stir to coat the vegetables.

Place on a large baking tray and bake on medium heat for 55 minutes.

Special tip: You can make a large batch of this dish and freeze individual serves to use through the week as an easy accompaniment to lean meat, chicken or fish. That means your fresh vegetables can be cooked straight away so that nothing goes to waste.

Oriental Stir-fry

Ingredients: 120 g lean beef, chicken or prawns per person, 3 tablespoons of olive oil, a bottle of oyster sauce and your favourite mix of stir-fry vegetables: mushrooms, broccoli or broccolini, carrots, zucchini, onion or spring onions. Alternatively, there are some wonderful frozen stir-fry vegetable mixes that are just as nutritious.

Slice the beef or chicken into narrow strips, or peel your prawns. Wash, peel and thinly slice the vegetables. Spray a wok or frypan with cooking spray and heat. Add 1 tablespoon of olive oil and cook your vegetables until slightly tender. Put the vegetables aside, spray the frypan or wok with cooking spray, add 2 tablespoons of olive oil and add the beef, chicken or prawns. Toss frequently until cooked. Then add 3 tablespoons of oyster sauce, add the cooked vegetables and heat gently for 3 more minutes.

Special tip: This dish can be served by itself, or with half a cup of cooked rice per person. It can also be served with noodles, but be sure to choose the low calorie varieties.

Tomato and Onion Relish

Ingredients: 3 tomatoes, 2 onions, 2 tablespoons of breadcrumbs and ½ tablespoon of olive oil.

Wash, peel and chop the vegetables into tiny pieces. Combine and stir in a small casserole dish with the olive oil, breadcrumbs and some salt and pepper.

Bake in a microwave oven for 5 minutes. Stir the ingredients again, and then cook for 3 more minutes.

Special tip: This is very low in calories and can be used as an accompaniment to meat, fish or chicken. You don't need those rich creamy sauces anymore! Then add the leftovers to your sandwich to make it truly delicious. This dish will keep for several days in the refrigerator. You can also add mushrooms and/or a few canned or frozen corn kernels.

Tomato Vegetable Soup

Ingredients: 2 large tomatoes, 1 onion, 2 carrots, 200 g pumpkin, 1 zucchini, several shallots, 1 parsnip, 1 potato, 2 beef or chicken stock cubes and 1 can of chopped tomatoes.

Stir stock cubes in 1½ litres of boiling water until dissolved. Wash and chop the vegetables into small pieces. Place in a large pot, add the stock and a little more water and add the can of tomatoes. Flavour with salt and pepper, add more water to taste and boil until vegetables are soft.

Special tip: Store in the refrigerator or freeze individual portions. This is only about 20 calories per serve.

Zucchini Ratatouille

Ingredients: 2 tomatoes, 2 onions and 5 zucchini

Wash and chop the vegetables into small chunks. Combine in a bowl with 1 tablespoon of olive oil and 2 tablespoons of minced garlic. Stir to coat the vegetables.

Place on a baking tray and bake on medium heat for 55 minutes.

Traditional Roast Beef and Baked Vegetables

Ingredients: A small piece of lean roast beef, chicken or lamb, potatoes, pumpkin, sweet potato, and carrot.

Place lean beef or other meat in a covered casserole, or bake uncovered in an oven or barbecue until meat is cooked to taste. Serve with brown gravy made with instant gravy powder and boiling water.

Wash and chop the vegetables into large pieces. Spray both sides with cooking spray, place on a lightly sprayed baking tray and bake on medium heat for 1 hour.

Special tip: As you can see, losing weight doesn't mean you can't enjoy a traditional roast dinner. The method I've described uses almost no fat and has far less calories but still tastes just as good.

CHAPTER 12: EXERCISE

My sad exercise history

I used to hate exercise and I hated sport even more. Even now, I always announce that I'm the world's worst at sport and truly believe that it would be hard to find anyone more dreadful than me.

My sorry saga began long ago when I was a child. School sport and gym classes were an agony for me, and I loved nothing better than to sit on the sidelines or hold the end of a skipping rope so that I would not have to participate. I couldn't even master riding a bicycle or a horse. And I didn't learn to swim until I was sixteen years old, when a friend finally taught me how to float. Can you believe it?

Naturally, when the other kids at school chose their teams I was always the last person to be picked. I didn't fare a great deal better in those adult exercise classes that most people enjoy. I'm always the worst in the class and the one that the teacher, with the best of intentions, tries to help the most. That does nothing for my self-confidence so I avoid that sort of activity.

The only forms of exercise I did enjoy were occasional dancing classes and some very low-key exercise classes. I enjoyed short walks but would complain if I had to walk more than a couple of kilometres. It seemed like such a long distance!

And then about six years ago, everything changed. I'd been feeling unwell for quite a few weeks, but my doctor could find anything wrong with me. I passed every test with flying colours, so we decided that my problems were just due to anxiety, even though I really had nothing in my life to worry about it.

That was the turning point. I was tired of feeling ill and decided to improve things. First of all, I looked at my lifestyle. I decided to live life to the full and be more active. I determined that each day I would go for a walk and in the evening I would spend less time in front of the television. I would try to enjoy each day as much as I could, and note down whatever I had enjoyed. Spending time with my husband or children, sharing a coffee with someone, going for a walk in the outdoors, seeing a beautiful view, having a great meal, browsing the shops or seeing a good television show or movie were all things that I might record.

The biggest change was my approach to exercise. At that time, I was living in a house perched on a hill. Just above the street was a bush reserve with a long, wide path that was six kilometres long. Best of all, there were panoramic views of Canberra, so it was the perfect place to go for a walk.

My daughter came with me on the first evening and urged me on so that I completed a three-kilometre walk. I couldn't believe it! I had breathed some fresh air, seen beautiful views, and spent time with my daughter all at the same time. And meanwhile, I had done some exercise.

Of course, it had been a struggle. I needed to stop at regular intervals, complained when I had to walk up a small hill, and felt utterly exhausted. But I had done it and I was determined to keep walking every night and develop the stamina of a normal person.

Almost every night, or in the early morning on weekends, I kept walking that trail. After a few weeks I started to walk four kilometres. And slowly I began to walk at a faster, more confident pace and didn't need to stop unless I wanted to enjoy those lovely views for a moment. I didn't even need to take a water bottle with me. I was starting to feel like the person I wanted to become.

I felt energised instead of collapsing with exhaustion when I arrived home. After a few months I could almost feel a spring in my step as my muscles slowly became a little bit stronger. And some of the little aches and pains in my legs began to disappear. Even more important, I began to feel incredibly healthy. I had cured myself!

So what exercise do I do now? I still walk several kilometres a day, and it has become such an important part of my life that I would never give it up. I do a few stretching and strengthening exercises at home every day, but I don't go to any exercise classes or belong to a gym. And I'm not planning to trek through the Himalayas or run a marathon. My walks are more than enough for me.

Those walks have other benefits, too. While I'm walking I love to watch the scenery around me, the beautiful bushland and scenic views. It clears my head, helps me relax and soothes my soul. It helps me to think more clearly, resolving any issues that I have. And it's also fun and a great way to spend some time!

Exercise your way to the slender you

The most efficient and effective ways to become the slender you are to follow your healthy eating plan and also do some exercise. They're the two most important elements of The One Way Diet. But all you need to aim for is thirty minutes of exercise every day.

It's true that you can lose weight without exercise provided you stick religiously to your healthy eating plan. It's also true that you might lose some weight without a healthy eating plan, but only if you exercise frantically for several hours every day. And who has the time or desire to do that? Some people find that if they do some regular exercise for quite a few months without changing their diet they might lose one or two kilos.

What does all that really mean for you? It means that you can't lose weight unless you follow a healthy eating plan. That is the most important thing to remember. The second thing to remember is that you could lose weight without exercise, but if you do some exercise it will help you in the most amazing ways.

Exercise is like the beautiful and elaborate icing on a wedding cake. The cake is tasty without that icing and would do the job of feeding all the wedding guests. But when the icing and decorations are added it becomes something wonderful that we all want to photograph and then devour enthusiastically.

Imagine the head of a large company without an assistant, or a surgeon in an operating theatre without a trusted nurse to hand her the instruments at just the right time. That secretary and nurse are playing the same role that exercise will play in your weight loss journey. It will become indispensable because it has so many benefits.

Why is exercise so beneficial, and why will it help you to lose weight? First of all, exercise will burn up some calories. If you sit down for half an hour you will burn about 44 calories. Standing for half an hour will burn about 50 calories. Walking at a moderate pace for thirty minutes will burn about 75 calories. See the difference it can make? While you are exercising, you will have a faster metabolic rate.

More vigorous exercise burns even more calories. If you are doing more than an hour of exercise each day you will need to eat slightly more than 1,200 calories a day (or 1,500 calories a day for men) to supply your body with a bit more fuel.

When you exercise, your metabolic rate increases and burns more calories. When you finish exercising, your metabolic rate will stay higher for a short while, so you'll burn even more calories. And because you'll have more energy and stronger muscles, your resting metabolic rate will start to be a little bit higher all day long.

Exercise has all sorts of other benefits as well. It will improve your mood because it releases some special chemicals in the brain. It will increase your energy levels because your heart and lungs will work more efficiently to deliver oxygen and nutrients to all your tissues. Your bones and muscles will become much stronger and you will notice an energising spring in your step.

Scientists have discovered that exercising increases the production of good cholesterol and reduces the production of bad cholesterol. That helps keep your blood flowing smoothly and helps prevent strokes and heart attacks. Exercise helps many medical conditions, and as you get older it helps prevent Type 2 Diabetes, dementia and accidental falls. Imagine how your co-ordination, balance and self-confidence would increase if you walked or did some other exercise for half an hour each day?

Exercise helps you to sleep better and stops you feeling tired and out of shape. And best of all, exercise is fun. You might not think it's fun right now, but soon you will. You can exercise with a friend, relative or work colleague, so that it can be a social event. Or it can be a great time just for yourself. If you exercise outside you will breathe some fresh air, clear your head and enjoy your surroundings. It's a wonderful way to release your stress, soothe your soul and calm your mind.

When you look at all those great effects, you can probably see why a little bit of exercise will be such a great help on your journey to find the slender you. Think carefully about the person you long to be. Would spend most of their day sitting down? Is the slender you energetic and healthy? Are they keen to live life to the full? I'm sure you'll agree that they're the sort of person who'd do some regular exercise.

Remember that your transformation to become the slender you won't happen overnight. He or she won't suddenly enter the world like Superman emerging from a phone booth dressed in his costume and cape. You'll get there in small steady steps and with just a little bit of exercise your journey will be faster and you will begin to feel much more like that person.

If you've chosen to travel the journey to find the slender you, then you should try to do some regular exercise.

Find the exercise that's right for you

I'm sure that some of you are already very sporty and regularly attend exercise classes or your local gym. Perhaps you play golf, netball or tennis, or you love to jog and always sign up for the local fun run. Some of you might even be thinking of losing weight so that you can try to run a marathon. That's wonderful, and you can pat yourself on the back because you already do some exercise. Just remember to keep doing exactly what you're doing.

Some of you, though, might loathe the thought of exercise so much that you would rather be dipped in acid, boiled in oil or run over by a train. Or you might have just descended into bad habits and exercise is no longer a part of your life. Worst of all, perhaps you feel that you're so overweight you feel embarrassed to be seen going for a walk. We all understand that feeling, but that doesn't mean you can't start to get the exercise you need.

Doctors recommend that you exercise for thirty minutes, five times a week. That's all. Don't listen to anyone who tells you that you need to do more than that. That doesn't sound like much, does it? It really will make a great difference to your fitness levels and help you to lose weight. But first you need to get started.

First of all, you need to find the time. You need thirty minutes, five times a week. If you think you're too busy and can't spare thirty minutes, then have a look at your schedule. Could you get up earlier or change your activities through the day or in the evening? Is there a TV show you always watch that you could miss? Is there something you do now that you could cut out?

You can also divide the time in two and do fifteen minutes twice a day. Or perhaps you could just start with fifteen minutes and work up to thirty minutes.

Secondly, you need to choose the sort of exercise you would like to do. You can choose different activities, or stick with just one. You might like to join an exercise class and also go for a walk several times a week. Or you might decide to visit your local gym and see if you would like to sign up and visit several times a week.

Don't be afraid to try a few different things and if you decide you don't like an activity, move on to something else. We all get bored and need a change of routine. Just don't give up altogether!

What sort of activities could you do? The list is probably endless. You could try walking, jogging, bicycling or dancing. You could join any sort of exercise class, or follow an exercise class on TV or online. You could join a gym or try a new sport.

But what if you're embarrassed to be seen exercising, or are so unfit you don't know what to do or where to start? Don't despair. Start by walking around your own garden, or even inside your own home. Start with ten minutes a day for one week, and then increase it by five minutes each week. How does that sound? As your confidence increases, you could walk to the end of you street and back. Before you know it, you'll be taking a half hour walk nearly every day.

Just remember that if you combine your healthy eating plan with some exercise, you'll travel more quickly and efficiently on that journey to find the slender you. And all you need is a minimum of thirty minutes, five times a week.

CHAPTER 13: MAKE THE MOST OF YOUR METABOLISM

Metabolism Muddle

Are you in a metabolism muddle? Metabolism is a popular word these days and there are more theories than anyone can count about its role in weight loss. There are millions of articles on the Internet that contain that word, and new scientific research on the subject is emerging all the time.

There's highly technical scientific information that is difficult to understand. There are diet plans that have you cutting out food groups or eating at certain times of the day or in in an effort to boost your metabolism. There are lists of strange foods and magic formulas that turn you into the perfect fat-burning machine. And you can also read articles that tell you exactly how to exercise so that you burn fat and build muscle.

You wouldn't be the only one to think that it was all a bit confusing. Do you find it overwhelming and don't know what to believe? The most important thing for you to remember is that you should not worry too much about your metabolism and what it is doing. Just like breathing, it's one of those things that keeps on keeping on, with or without your help.

All you need to know is that if you follow a healthy eating plan and do some exercise then your metabolism will behave quite well most of the time and keep on burning those calories at a reasonable pace. Your metabolism will stay in the good zone and help you to lose weight.

If your weight loss slows down a bit, then it's probably because your metabolism has entered a bad zone and just needs a bit of stirring up. You can boost it by doing a few more minutes of exercise each day, and I'll talk more about that in the chapter about perilous plateaus. That will kick your metabolism into the good zone, and away you go again travelling on that journey to find the slender you.

The perfect metabolism

I've talked about a good zone and a bad zone for your metabolism. But is there a perfect zone? Would it be possible to have the perfect metabolism for weight loss?

A score of one hundred percent in any competition or test is usually regarded as perfect. But absolute perfection is very hard to describe and it can be even harder to find. When it comes to human beings, there are few of us who would claim to be perfect, and individual opinions on perfection can vary widely. Occasionally, there's an article in the media about someone who supposedly has the perfect face or perfect body. But when it comes to our character then perfection is much harder to attain.

The perfect metabolism doesn't exist, but if you think about what it might be like then you'll understand your own metabolism a little bit better. It's just like watching a video of an expert with the perfect golf swing. You know you'll never get close to playing golf like that, but you can try to emulate them to a small extent.

You know that your metabolism is your fuel consumption rate. That's how fast your body burns calories, just like your car's fuel consumption rate. You also know that your body uses glucose for fuel. When the glucose levels in your bloodstream drop, your body uses its two reserve tanks to supply fuel. First it uses up glycogen, and then it uses up your fat reserves. Both of these are converted to glucose.

If you had the perfect metabolism your body would steadily burn your fat reserves twenty-four hours a day to help you lose weight. You would lose exactly the same amount of weight each day, and even every hour, all through your weight loss journey. If you graphed your daily weight loss, it would be a straight line until you reached your goal weight and found the slender you.

Just imagine some lucky person called Mary, who had an almost-perfect metabolism that helped her to lose weight for twenty-four hours every day. All day long, the glucose levels in Mary's blood stream remain steady.

She eats a tiny amount of food all day long, but fewer calories than her body needs. Every time she eats, her glucose levels rise ever so slightly and then gradually drop. When her body needs more glucose, the glycogen reserves get used up, followed by her fat reserves. While she's asleep, her body still needs glucose to function and so her body keeps the fuel levels constant, burning up more of her fat reserves. I can almost see her lying on the pillow, asleep but smiling at her never-failing weight loss.

That, unfortunately, is the stuff of fantasy. Your metabolism can never achieve that state of perfection. The glucose levels will always rise and fall in your blood stream throughout the day, and your body will do its best to hang on to your fat reserves in case there is a famine.

All you can do is try to keep your metabolism working steadily for as many hours a day as possible. It will never reach perfection, but you might be able to give your metabolism a score of good or very good, and you don't want it to behave badly, slow down and stop you losing weight.

Keep your metabolism in the good zone

The One Way Diet, with its focus on healthy eating and a small amount of exercise, is designed to help keep your metabolism in the good zone. If you eat the right sorts of food six times a day and also try to do at least thirty minutes of exercise five times a week, you'll help to boost your metabolism. You don't want your metabolism to slow down and slip into the bad zone where it tries to slow down your weight loss.

With the healthy eating plan, you eat six times throughout the day, from breakfast until an hour or two before bedtime. Most of your food is complex carbohydrates plus some protein and a tiny amount of fat, and includes fruit and vegetables. Your body needs about 2,000 calories for normal maintenance, but for effective weight loss you consume about 1,200 calories a day (or 1,500 calories a day for a man).

Because you're taking in complex carbohydrates all day long, your blood glucose levels stay fairly steady for twenty-four hours a day. But because you're eating fewer calories than you need for maintenance your body uses up those reserve tanks of fuel to boost the levels of glucose in your blood. First it will use those easy-to-access supplies of glycogen. When they get depleted, it will start to burn your fat reserves.

When you do some exercise your body is doing more work, so it will need more glucose. It burns up that fuel more quickly for about an hour after you finish exercising. As your muscles become stronger over a long period of time, your baseline body metabolism will be boosted.

Both your healthy eating plan and exercise program help to keep your metabolism in the good zone. The finer scientific details about your body's metabolism can be left to the experts to worry about, while you focus on the great adventure that lies before you. Your metabolism will keep chugging along, and slowly your excess fat reserves will disappear.

One day, you'll stand on those bathroom scales and realise that you've achieved your dream.

CHAPTER 14: TIPS FOR COPING WITH EACH DAY

A new approach to shopping

Deep inside your brain you can find all the tools for survival that you need on your weight loss journey. You believe that you will find the slender you, and all along your journey there are exciting mini-goals to reach. You know you'll look and feel amazing at those big events you're looking forward to in a few months time, and you can't wait.

But as you know, daily life can be tedious, and to cope with your new healthy eating plan you need a few practical tips to increase your chance of successfully finishing the journey. Just imagine going on a vacation and forgetting your walking shoes, your swimming costume and your toiletries. They're the little details that don't figure in your dreams about the trip, but they're basic necessities that are essential.

The first basic necessity to think about is shopping. If you tend to shop every day on your way home, or you only run to the supermarket when your pantry is bare, then you might have to change your ways just a little bit. If you open your pantry or refrigerator and grab anything you see, or if your pantry is full of chocolate cookies and chips, then you definitely need to have a serious talk to yourself.

First of all, look inside your pantry and refrigerator. If there are foods that will tempt you to stray from your healthy eating plan then throw them out, give them away or put them somewhere else. I know you might have other people in the house, but make a decision about whether those foods are beneficial for them. None of us can resist the look of that pack of cookies or chips, but if they're not on the shelf then you can't eat them late one night when you've had a rough day. They may have cost you some money, but you are worth far more than that.

Then start to stock your pantry with all those great, healthy foods that you'll be eating from now on. You don't ever want to get up in the morning and find there's no healthy food for breakfast, or skim milk in the fridge. You don't want to go to work without the food you need for your snacks and lunch. And you don't want to find that you're missing those ingredients you need for a healthy dinner.

Before you venture out to do your shopping, you need to write a list of everything you need to buy, including fruit and vegetables, skim milk, no-fat yoghurts and lean serves of protein foods like meat. That way, you won't forget anything and you'll be less tempted to stray into the realms of impulse buying.

When you reach the supermarket, stick faithfully to your shopping list and check the labels on any packaging to be sure that you're really buying a good, low calorie item for your healthy eating plan. Yoghurt is the perfect example of why it's helpful to read those food labels. No-fat varieties can be about 60 calories for a small tub, but a low-fat variety can be about 120 calories. Always check labels or refer to a calorie counter book or website to be certain about the calorie content of everything you eat.

Buy food in small packages if you think that you'll be tempted to over-eat if you buy a large economy size. When it comes to buying meat, make sure it's as lean as possible and just the right amount for you and your family.

Don't ever be tempted to impulse buy those foods that aren't in your healthy eating plan. If you really find it an emotional struggle to go to the supermarket, then ask someone to shop for you, or make sure you don't go near the aisles that tempt you to stray.

Eat six times a day

The second basic necessity is to eat six times a day. That means breakfast, lunch and dinner plus a snack mid-morning, mid-afternoon and evening. Regular eating will help to keep your metabolism in the good zone, steadily burning up your fat reserves. Don't be tempted to skip breakfast or any other meal.

I know how easy it is to become busy or so involved in an activity that it becomes difficult to have that snack or meal at just the right time. That's why it's important to plan ahead and always make sure you have a snack with you.

If your friends are meeting for coffee and cake, or there is a morning tea at work, pack your own snack and have it with the rest of the group or, if you feel uncomfortable doing that, eat it in private. Don't be shy about refusing a slice of that lovely cake your friend has made: your friends or associates will accept that you're trying to lose weight. You can still enjoy a cup of coffee. If you have an activity in the evening, take your own snack along in a little snack bag. Your friends will envy your self-control and be happy to help in any way they can.

Snacks

The third basic necessity is to think of some healthy snacks. We're all familiar with organising meals, but planning snacks might be something new for you.

You know that you need three snacks a day, and they should contain less than about 100 calories each. You might have noticed that my favourite evening snack is just a bit more than that. You can create all sorts of wonderful snacks for yourself as long as you carefully count the calories, but I'd like to make a few suggestions to get you started.

Fresh or frozen fruit and vegetables are the perfect snack because they generally contain fibre, keep you satisfied for quite a while and have good nutrients to increase your health. You could try a piece of fruit or some berries, such as blueberries and strawberries. Vegetables are delicious, and you can dip them in a small amount of hummus or salsa dip. You could make a batch of Vegetable soup and have it with some rice crackers or bread.

If you carefully check the calorie count, you could eat a few nuts or a small amount of dried fruit. You could have a piece of cheese, a hard-boiled egg, or a fat-free yoghurt.

There are some biscuits that are low in calories, particularly plain sweet biscuits. Check the labels very carefully. They won't keep you satisfied for very long, though, so you need to regard them as an occasional treat, or at least have no more than one or two biscuits a day.

Invent your own great low-calorie snacks and never be tempted to skip a snack in an effort to reduce your calories. They're an essential part of your healthy eating plan.

Portion Sizes

The fourth basic necessity is to carefully watch your portion sizes. You may have become accustomed to filling your plate as if it's your last meal on the planet Earth. Just remember that your stomach is only about the size of your clenched fist. That's all the amount of food you need to consume. Once you've become accustomed to eating less you'll wonder why you ever piled your plate so high.

Have you ever heard of the expression, "eating like a bird"? You might have some friends with slender figures and small appetites. Do you think that the slender you eats like a bird as well? To become the slender you, that person deep within your mind who is screaming to get out, take up the challenge of eating like a bird and carefully check your portion sizes. Soon that will be second nature to you. However, always eat at least 1,200 calories a day (or 1,500 calories for a man).

Try to invest in a little set of digital kitchen scales if you don't already have one. Measure everything you can at first to make sure your portions are the right size, especially for meat and fish. In some cases, you'll be pleasantly surprised, but in others cases you'll realise that you need to be careful. Take peanut butter, for instance: one tablespoon is fine, but if you pile it a centimetre thick on your slice of toast then you'll need to cut back.

It won't be long before you think those smaller portion sizes are quite normal and just a part of the way you live your life.

Water

The fifth basic necessity is water. Water, in some form, is an essential part of your daily diet. It's vital for your survival, and as we hear all the time we can survive for only a few days without it. Luckily, though, we're not all stuck in the middle of the Sahara Desert and we don't have to drink litres of water every day.

Provided that you have a few cups of fluid each day, you'll give your body everything it needs to burn off those fat reserves. Naturally, if you're doing some vigorous exercise or you're in a very hot climate, you might want to drink a bit more. Water, tea, coffee and diet soft drinks (sodas) are all virtually calorie free. You can also include soup as part of your fluid consumption.

Avoid those drinks that are high in calories because they're packed with sugar: any form of alcohol, normal soft drinks (sodas), juices and cordials. You could include an occasional glass of wine or beer in your healthy eating plan, but carefully monitor the calories.

You may have a medical condition that means you shouldn't drink too much fluid. Make sure you ask your doctor about how much fluid you can safely drink each day, and carefully follow their advice.

Armed with some knowledge about those basic necessities for your survival, you'll soon be travelling successfully on that journey to find the slender you.

CHAPTER 15: THE PERILOUS PLATEAU

The definition of a plateau

You've probably heard of a weight loss plateau, but what does it really mean? A geologist will tell you that a plateau is an elevated, level expanse of land raised sharply above the surrounding landscape on at least one side. If you trek along the Tibetan Plateau, which is one of the great plateaus of the world, then you'll walk for a long time along fairly level ground. That plateau is one thousand kilometres long, two-and-a-half thousand kilometres wide, and extremely cold. It's so vast and high that it's called the roof of the world.

Have you ever seen the Blue Mountains west of Sydney? It's a stunning example of a plateau edged by steep cliffs. When you stand at one of the famous scenic lookouts, you're standing right on the edge of a plateau.

I'm afraid that the word *plateau* has also come to have another meaning of significance to those who want to lose weight. Sometimes, that word is used to describe a state of little or no change after a time of activity or progress.

Just imagine that champion swimmer who dreams of winning an Olympic gold medal. He has a new coach with a great training program and for several weeks his personal best time is decreasing. He's improving so much that he thinks he might be selected for the next world championships. But then his performance reaches a plateau. His speed doesn't improve for several weeks, and he begins to doubt his own ability to get any better. Worst of all, he wonders if he'll ever achieve his dream.

Remember that this champion swimmer is not just taking a rest. He's training just as hard, swimming up and down the pool every day, working out in the gym and taking his coach's advice. His experience is an example of that second meaning of the word *plateau*.

You are just like that champion swimmer, working hard each day to reach your next mini-goal and achieve that final dream of finding the slender you. Everything you do on your journey is similar to that swimmer's training program. Your healthy eating plan, your exercise program and your strong motivation are all helping you to achieve your dream. You can make good progress most of the time. But sometimes, just like any champion athlete, you can reach a plateau where your progress seems to stall or slow down.

You might have been losing weight steadily for two months. Happy days! And then, the next week, you stand on the bathroom scales. Your weight is the same, or only 100 grams lower. The following week, it still hasn't changed much. You don't seem to have lost any weight. That could last a couple of weeks or perhaps longer.

The worst thing about a plateau is that makes you feel demoralised and unhappy. You start to doubt your ability to complete your weight loss journey. You begin to wonder if your healthy eating plan is really working and you're tempted to give up. You might even think that you are meant to be overweight!

That's why a plateau is so perilous.

The good news is that a weight loss plateau can be conquered quickly and you are going to learn how take on that challenge.

Why does it happen?

First of all, before you learn how to conquer the perilous plateau with all the courage and skill of a mountain climber, you need to understand the possible causes. Can you imagine a doctor trying to treat you without understanding what was wrong with you? There are several reasons why your weight loss might stall after several weeks or months of success.

First of all, remember the effect of your ancient ancestors. Your body is trying to conserve your fat reserves so that you can survive that long cold winter without much food. It doesn't want you to lose weight. After a couple of months of wonderful progress with your weight loss, your body's metabolism, the rate it burns calories, might slow down a bit in an attempt to conserve your fat reserves.

Have you been eating less than 1,200 calories a day (or 1,500 calories for a man)? If so, then your body might think that you're in starvation mode and is trying very hard to slow down. Don't be tempted to starve yourself like that because the next thing you know your weight loss will stall. That will be disheartening when you've been restricting your diet so much.

Have you started to do some exercise? If you haven't, and especially if your lifestyle is very sedentary, then your metabolism might be running on low gear. It might have become used to your diet and needs a bit of a boost, a foot on the accelerator, to start burning those fat reserves again.

The second reason that your weight loss might stall is that you may be eating too many calories. How can that be, if you've been on a healthy eating plan of 1,200 calories or just a bit more? There are a couple of reasons for that, and sometimes they can work in combination with each other to produce a double whammy effect.

The first reason is that you might be eating more calories each day than you realised. Perhaps one day when you went out or entertained, you over-indulged and ate more calories than you thought you did. Then it has sabotaged your weight loss for a week. I'm going to talk more about that in the chapters on eating out and surviving vacations.

Just imagine that you've been following your healthy eating plan for a while and have stopped meticulously counting your calories. You might also have added one or two extra things to your daily diet, or increased your portions slightly. Perhaps you're eating something that isn't as low in calories as you thought. You might find that if you carefully add up all your calories each day then they add up to more than you realised.

The second reason for eating too many calories might be that you have lost weight and your body doesn't need as many calories. You're thinner than you were and because there is a smaller body to maintain you need fewer calories to do it. It's just the same as needing less petrol for a smaller car.

I'm not saying that you should eat less than 1,200 calories. You should never do that. But if you're eating more than that, then you might need to eat a bit less to keep on losing weight successfully every week.

Now think what might happen if you combine all those effects. You don't get much exercise, you add a few more calories to your healthy eating plan, and you become thinner so you don't need as many calories for your body's maintenance requirements. You've been making great progress on that wonderful journey to find the slender you, but then you stand on the bathroom scales and find that your weight is stalling.

How to conquer that perilous plateau

What should you do if you suddenly find yourself standing right in the middle of a perilous plateau? One thing you must never, ever do is become upset, and you must never think of giving up. Just remember that you will emerge at the other end of that plateau and you will carry on making great progress along your weight loss journey. You will become that slender you.

All it will take to get to the other side is a little bit more effort. Just imagine that you're in a small car travelling slowly along the road in low gear.

You need to go a bit faster. So what will you do? Just press your foot on the accelerator a bit harder. Hey presto: your car starts to speed up and you're making better progress on that journey.

Remember that swimming champion who had reached a plateau in his swimming speed after making steady progress for a few weeks? If you were his coach, what would you tell him to do? The last thing I would claim to be is a swimming coach, but my suggestion would be that he adds some more exercises to his training program. Perhaps that will do the trick and his performance will show some improvement.

You may have found yourself on a perilous plateau because your body wanted to tell you that a little readjustment was necessary. All it will take is some very small changes to kick-start your weight loss once again.

First and easiest of all to think about is exercise. If you haven't started to do any, then re-read the chapter on exercise and begin, ever so slightly at first, to do some exercise and increase your metabolism. The wonderful thing is that it will also make you feel good by elevating your mood and soothing your mind and soul.

If you're already doing some exercise then increase your effort slightly. If you walk for thirty minutes, increase it by five or ten minutes. That boost might be all you need to get your metabolism stirred up and zooming along so that it helps you to lose weight once again.

Make sure that you haven't dropped below 1,200 calories a day (or 1,500 calories for a man). Your body might have gone into starvation mode and that's why your weight loss has stalled. If that is happening to you, increase those calories and try to stir up your body with a little bit of exercise.

Carefully count the calories that you're consuming every day. If you've been eating more than 1,200 calories (or 1,500 calories for a man), then you might need to cut back a little bit or be very careful about what you eat for a week or two. Keep in mind that if you're much thinner, your body might need fewer calories for daily maintenance. But never, ever go lower than 1,200 calories a day.

If you're following the healthy eating plan and doing some exercise then your journey along that perilous plateau should be very short. Soon, you'll make some progress and you're on the way once again in search of the slender you.

CHAPTER 16: CLOTHES AND MORE CLOTHES

Black trousers and four-man tents: my history with fashion

You're on that journey to find the slender you and one of the most exciting aspects about that journey will be your clothes. For so long, some of you have kept your body hidden under loose clothing, hoping that no one would notice those extra lumps and bumps. You've forgotten what it's like to dress so that you feel sensational. For quite a while, you haven't looked forward to shopping for clothes or showing off your outfit on a night out. But now, the time is at hand for you to shine.

First, though, I want to talk about my own fashion history. I hope my story might have some similarities to yours and that my suggestions might help you.

I'm afraid to admit that, previously, I had a closet full of clothes in widely varying sizes. I suppose you could say that I had several sets of clothes to fit all the different sizes I became as I gained weight and lost weight. I would buy something I liked and, much to my disappointment, promptly start to grow out of it. My bedroom closet had spilled over into a couple of old suitcases and a few cardboard boxes full of clothes that I could no longer squeeze into. It was very frustrating, and I would marvel at people I knew who stayed the same size throughout their adult lives.

I know the feeling of trying to squeeze into a pair of trousers that I wore last season, and finding that they're just a bit too tight to wear this year. Thank goodness most trousers these days have some elastane to give them a small amount of stretch - I've often been in desperate need of it.

The mainstays of my wardrobe were loose trousers in black or other dark colours and baggy tops that covered my hips. Jackets were often voluminous and flowing, with enough fabric to make a four-man tent. The main objective, or so I thought, was to hide and flatter my body as much as I could.

At my fattest, I didn't want to buy any clothes because my plan was always to lose weight. So I wore the same few ghastly items again and again. Whenever I did shop for clothes, I needed to choose from the large size racks or go to stores specialising in big sizes. And it was never easy to find something that fitted my body properly. I have a small bust and it seemed that larger-size clothes were always made for women with a large bust, big shoulders, long arms and long legs.

Trying on clothes was never the fun experience that it's meant to be. Inside those tiny fitting room booths with my body close to a mirror, my confidence sank at the sight of all my flesh. The experience became even more depressing when I couldn't fit into an item, as so often happened.

Then, at last, everything changed. I gradually lost all my excess weight, and had some great style advice from my beautiful daughter.

Experience taught me some simple fashion rules to follow when you're on a weight loss journey. They're not the sorts of rules that are essential. But if you try some of them, then I'm sure you'll discover that the journey to find the slender you will become more exciting and much more fun!

Gentlemen, these rules also apply to you. The time has come for you to discard those giant tops and trousers and find out how you can dress to impress.

Dress to impress on your weight loss journey

There's nothing more exciting than fitting into smaller size clothes. If you've never experienced that thrill, then brace yourself because you are in for treat. First of all, settle in to your weight loss journey and focus on your healthy eating plan and exercise. You have enough to keep you busy in those early weeks. But after a month has passed it will be time to think about your clothing and that will be just the motivation you need at that point.

First, let's start with your current wardrobe. Perhaps some of you don't have clothes in any smaller sizes. But others might have quite a few items in the back of their closet or stored in a box. Now's the time to get them all out and spend an afternoon sorting through everything.

There might be items you know you'd never wear again, and you wonder what you were thinking when you bought them. There might be items so old and stained that they need to be thrown out. Be careful, though. Don't throw out an item just because it looks too small and you don't know how it would ever fit you again. You might surprise yourself.

Now, separate your clothes into different sizes. Hopefully, you now have a series of garments for every step along your weight loss journey. Try some on and take some photos, just so you have a record of how they fail to fit you now. You'll almost fit into some items, and others will seem impossibly small. But you will get there! Then store those clothes somewhere handy so that you can try them on again in a few weeks' time.

When you've lost a few more kilos, you can try on those outfits that were close to fitting you and see how they look. A pair of jeans might not get past your thighs. But in a month or two you might be able to pull them all the way up. A month or two later, you might be able to do up the zipper. Can you imagine how fantastic that will feel? That's the perfect way to demonstrate how much weight you've lost.

After a few months of weight loss, you will surprise yourself. The clothes you're currently wearing will become too big and you'll decide to put them away out of sight. That jacket you couldn't do up now fastens easily and fits you perfectly. The clothes you couldn't squeeze into are starting to become your regular wardrobe. And you know that each day you're getting closer to fitting into those much smaller sizes.

The outfits you're trying on in those smaller sizes may not be your current choice for fashion. There might be items that are so old that they're totally out of date. That doesn't matter, though. It's a thrill just to know that you can fit into them again. Later on, if you no longer want them, you can place them in the charity bin. Be cautious, though, because retro fashion is all the rage and something you think went out of fashion in the eighties or nineties might be the latest look. Mixing and matching vintage pieces is also popular, and could become a new hobby of yours as you re-discover the joys of fashion.

But what should you do if you don't have any smaller sizes? Perhaps you've been the same weight for so long that the clothes in your current size are all you have. I have a few friends like that, and I've watched them lose weight while still wearing their large baggy outfits. I told one friend who was losing weight that her trousers would fall down soon unless she either bought a smaller pair or bought some braces to hold them up.

It's easy to understand why you wouldn't want to buy new garments that would only fit you for a few weeks as you travel on your weight loss journey. Clothes are expensive, and we usually want to get plenty of wear out of them. Sadly, though, if you keep wearing your big baggy fashions, then you are missing out on half the fun of losing weight and your motivation will be harder to maintain.

Your dress size will drop every time you lose about six or eight kilograms. Just say that you are currently size twenty. When you've lost about 20 kilograms, you might be a size fourteen. Just imagine it! But if you're still wearing those baggy, size-twenty trousers and T-shirts, then you're keeping your weight loss hidden from everyone, including yourself. Somewhere under those large clothes that are draped on your body like heavy curtains, you have a much smaller body.

Now put on some size 14 trousers with a tailored waistband. And put on a slim fitted blouse. Look in a full-length mirror and be completely stunned. Your outfit flatters you and shows just how slim you are. It shows your figure to the best advantage. You can see how wonderful you look and so can everyone else.

Try to dress in clothes that fit the new you at every step of the way. Forget your old ideas about loose, voluminous clothing. Whatever your size, wear clothes that are made to fit you. You'll actually notice how great you look and how slim you've become.

I know that most of us don't have a fortune to spend on buying new clothes, and we certainly can't buy a closet full of clothes every two months while our size keeps falling. That's why so many of us keep wearing our old baggy clothes for as long as we can. But if you don't have a wardrobe that already has some smaller-sized clothes, what can you do?

There are some fantastic ways to keep you always dressed in the right size on that journey to find the slender you. First of all, there are your friends, family, colleagues and neighbours, who might lend or give you some of their old clothes. You could even suggest a swap party, where people bring along those items they'd like to exchange. You can have fun together and get some new clothes at the same time.

You can shop at vintage or thrift stores that always sell a wide range of items. Most of those stores have some great quality clothes for just a few dollars, and you'll be amazed at the incredible fashion labels you can find. You can launder them when you get home and they'll be almost like new. You'll also be helping the charity each time you make a purchase.

So, you see, there really are no excuses for staying in those baggy over-sized clothes of yours. Enjoy every moment of the journey to find the slender you by dressing to impress both yourself and others.

The joy of dressing the slender you

You've worked so hard and finally you're getting very close to finding the slender you. You can walk proudly past those fashion stores for large ladies or men and those stands in department stores with signs like *large is lovely* and *real women.* They used to be your fashions, but not any more.

Can you imagine how deliriously wonderful it will be when you can walk into a store like that and find that nothing in there that will fit you? And it will feel even better to walk into a trendy fashion store and find a skinny shop assistant who is keen to help you. Savour every moment as you choose a few things to try on.

You can visit all those boutiques and online sites selling gorgeous clothes for people just like you. Someone who isn't overweight! Now is the time to discover the wonder of all those beautiful fashions out there. And it's also time to show the world your new figure. It's doesn't matter how old you are, the moment has arrived to dress like the slender you.

I've already talked about some ways to find clothes at very low cost. Now, after that long journey, you can finally invest in a few items that make you look terrific.

Now that you're slim, you don't need to wear loose comfortable trousers and long loose tops. And you don't need to wear black trousers with an elasticised waist. I'm sure that you have excuses for sticking with clothes like that. You might think that you're too old to look fashionable, or you're so accustomed to covering up your body that you find it strange to wear something tighter. You might even think that you wouldn't be comfortable in clothes that weren't loose. If that's what you think, then you're wrong on all counts.

Perhaps you're not quite sure how to go about putting your new wardrobe together. And perhaps you don't realise how fantastic you can look for very little effort. In fact, it takes just as much effort to dress fashionably and look great as it does to dress dowdily in loose clothes. I've already talked about ways to get some new clothes at very little cost. Now I want to give you a few simple fashion tips to make you look as fantastic as you feel. And that applies to men as well!

The very first requirement is to find the colours that suit you best, and complement your hair and skin tones.

There are several ways to find the best palette of colours for you. You can research that topic on the Internet, or go to the library to find a book on the subject. Get a friend to help you if you're not sure. When you find a list of colours that suit you, try some fabrics against your skin and see if you like them. I bet you'll be surprised at how nice you look in the right tones. And you might be amazed to find that some of the colours you've favoured for a long time don't really suit you at all.

The same principles apply to men. Choose masculine tones from the palette of colours that suit you best, and you'll be surprised how your appearance will be enhanced.

Now that you're choosing the right colours, the next fashion tip is to accessorise. You could be wearing a simple pair of trousers and a top. But if you add a belt, some earrings and a necklace, then you are starting to create a great outfit. Better yet, wear a scarf and some bangles to instantly transform your outfit. Men could add a nice belt, a smart pair of shoes, and a vest, scarf or jacket. You can get some inspiration by looking at fashion photos online or the displays in store windows.

The third fashion tip is to co-ordinate your outfit so that the colours and pieces you're wearing all blend together well. The fourth and final tip is to browse the fashion boutiques and vintage or thrift stores. Try on plenty different items, just to see how they look. Don't have any preconceived ideas about what suits you. When you try on something unusual, you might get a very pleasant surprise. Take a thorough look in that dressing room mirror, see how you look from every angle, and make sure what you've chosen is in a colour that suits you.

Whatever you do purchase, always make sure it's something that makes you look great and don't compromise. If it's the right style but the wrong colour, or vice versa, then just leave it. There are plenty of other clothes out there.

You've worked so hard to find the slender you, and now you can finally enjoy all those fashions. With a small amount of effort, you can show the world how wonderful you look.

CHAPTER 17: EATING OUT

The challenge of eating out

Just imagine a ship loaded with cargo for delivery to a final destination. If only the captain could sail there without any delays, he'd finish his journey rapidly. But he's been told he has to stop at several ports along the way, and each time he stops he loses time. The journey takes much longer than expected, and the captain feels very frustrated.

What's even worse, those ports he needs to visit are dangerous, with rocks, reefs and other hazards. He could easily hit those snags and the ship might founder, so he has to be very vigilant throughout the voyage.

That's what your journey to find the slender you might be like if you dine out frequently without taking some special precautions. You're keen to travel that journey every single day to find the slender you. It's not too difficult when you're able to prepare your meals at home, carefully cooking the low-fat way and counting the calories of everything you prepare.

But it's much more difficult when you dine out, and you need to be just as careful with your menu choices as that captain when he sails into those dangerous ports. Try adding up the calories in some of your favourite choices and see how those dishes could sabotage your valiant efforts to stay on course with a 1,200-calorie diet (or 1,500 calories for a man).

Does that mean you need to stay home and avoid restaurants and cafes until you finish your journey and find the slender you? Do you need to ignore your friends and family and stop all your normal social activities? No, of course you don't. But you do need to adopt a new approach to eating out so that your journey is not delayed any more than you would like.

When I was in my early twenties, dining out was a rare event and considered to be quite a treat. These days, many people eat out several times a week and there's a wide range of options to choose from. It's become a part of our regular weekly lifestyle and because it's so hard to avoid, advice about making healthy choices is an important part of most weight loss programs.

I love eating out and could once be counted on to choose a calorie-laden main course and dessert. And a starter as well! Every Saturday morning I enjoyed coffee and a cupcake in my favourite patisserie. And when I took my first cruise, a two-week voyage around New Zealand, I indulged in all the courses available at dinner, not to mention the other meals, with no consideration of the calorie content. It's no wonder my weight was on an upward spiral.

Everybody has a different lifestyle, and that certainly applies to eating out. Some of you might dine out rarely, while others eat out every day. Some people go to a restaurant once a week, or meet with friends or relatives for a regular meal. Dining out can include a visit to a café or a lunch outing, as well as dinner. It can also include those daily visits to a fast food restaurant to grab some takeaway lunch or a late meal after an exhausting day at work. Frequently, it includes a glass or two (or more) of alcohol.

Some of you might be required to dine out as part of your work. You might work long hours, travelling around and grabbing food on the run as you go. Or your work might include a round of socialising or events that include eating opportunities. If you have a demanding job like that, you'll find it difficult to organise your lifestyle to suit your healthy eating plan.

But there is a solution. Now is the time, before you start your journey, to rethink your approach to eating out. There are a few key strategies that you can adopt to help you cope.

The first thing to think about is drinking. One glass of wine or beer is quite okay, provided that you count the calories in your daily total. But it will be very difficult to stick to the healthy eating plan if you drink any more than that.

So what can you do? Try to have a diet soft drink (soda) or iced water after you finish your first drink, or replace it with a cup of coffee, and you'll manage to stay on that weight loss journey to find the slender you. If you can reduce that to one glass per week, your health will benefit and your journey will be much smoother.

If your friends or relatives ask what you're doing, tell them that you're on a strict diet. They'll probably be very understanding and want to help you as much as they can. I know it might seem very hard at first to say no to those extra drinks, but you'll soon get used to it. And when you stand on those scales and see your weight loss, you'll feel so good that you won't mind missing out on a drink or two.

The second thing to think about is your attitude to eating out. Try not to think of every dining out experience as a decadent indulgence. If you only eat out once every six months, it would be okay to choose the most tempting items on the menu, drowning in calories. But if you dine out more frequently than that, indulging in those foods will stop you reaching your final destination.

Think of eating out as a regular part of life that you can carefully manage in order to achieve your goals. Always keep the slender you in the forefront of your mind, and remember that you're on a journey to find that incredible person. Then you won't mind missing out on that fattening dessert or making a different choice for your main course.

If you succumb to temptation one evening, don't despair. We all do that. It's not a problem because you simply need to resume your weight loss journey on the next day and hopefully in the following week your weight loss will be better. Don't ever become discouraged or tempted to give up or because of one day or night of overeating. You are going to complete your journey!

The third thing to think about is what to select in any restaurant or café. It's time to take control of your menu choices so that you can eat out, have a wonderful time, but still continue on your weight loss journey.

So what menu items should you choose? Your goal is to avoid items that are fried or battered, or items that contain cheese, cream, bacon, salad dressings, sour cream or cream cheese. Avoid fancy sauces and items that are cooked in butter. Avoid breads because they'll add to your calories. And try not to choose fast food restaurants because many of their menu choices contain high levels of fat and sugar.

Now at last for what you *can* eat and enjoy! You can order salads without dressing, grilled vegetables or a baked potato without sour cream. Choose a main course of grilled, poached, barbecued or baked meat, fish or chicken. Ask for sauces on the side, and eat only a tiny amount. Stir-fries with boiled rice are also a great choice.

You can enjoy mustard, herbs and spices, lemon juice, tomato sauce, horseradish or salsa as condiments. If you're eating out for breakfast, you can choose poached eggs on toast (with no butter) or an omelette with tomato and onion. And if you're meeting a friend for coffee, bring your normal snack and eat that while enjoying a coffee, or eat it before you get there.

If you're buying a sandwich, ask for it to be served with no butter or margarine. Have one slice of meat or cheese and plenty of salad without dressing. Beware of soups and elaborate sandwiches because they can contain far more calories than you'd realise.

Portion sizes are the fourth and final thing to think about. Remember to eat only a small serve whenever you eat out.

I'm sure you've already noticed that restaurants and cafes often serve much larger portions than you need. Some eateries even specialise in giant servings. You might make a great diet-conscious choice, but if the restaurant serves a massive portion you're eating two or three times the calories!

Luckily, you know that your stomach is only the size of a fist and you understand the importance of small portion sizes. So what can you do if you're given a portion size that would feed a Tyrannosaurus?

There are two simple solutions. Firstly, when you're ordering, you can try asking for a small serve. Hopefully, that will work and they might even charge you less.

The second solution is to eat just a fraction of the serving that you're given. If you're handed a large piece of steak, only eat a part of it. You'll enjoy it and feel great because you know that you're sticking to your healthy eating plan. You won't notice that you haven't eaten the entire serve, because you've had a reasonable taste and thoroughly enjoyed it.

Don't be afraid to ask for the options you're seeking or too shy to ask for an item to be served without the sauce or with a salad. If a restaurant wants your custom, they'll be happy to oblige - and you'll be even happier, knowing that you'll lose weight that week.

Explore low-calorie options for each type of cuisine

Most people like to visit some international restaurants these days. Chinese, Thai, Indian, Italian, French and Mexican restaurants are common. If you have some favourite international eateries, it's easy to compile a list of good choices for each of those. And that list can travel with you wherever you go so that you're always prepared.

Everyone loves their favourite Asian restaurant for an easy meal or takeaway, and it's one of the best choices for that weight loss journey. Choose a soup or a stir-fry with plenty of vegetables and some lean chicken or beef. Try to avoid fried or battered dishes and dishes with thick sweet sauces. Beware of those fried entrees: they seem small but they have plenty of calories.

Most of us love an occasional curry at an Indian restaurant. Try to choose curries with a vegetable or lentil base, steamed vegetables and dry tandoori dishes. Stay well away from those curries made with coconut milk, and fried entrees covered in batter.

French restaurants are full of tempting treats. Try to choose steamed or grilled seafood, salad with vinaigrette dressing, French bread, steamed vegetables or a small serve of lean meat with a wine-based sauce. You can also choose sorbets or fruit. Try to avoid creamy sauces and desserts.

There are many calories lurking in Italian restaurants but you should be able to find some good choices. Select minestrone soup, pasta with marinara sauces and a sorbet. Try to avoid lasagne, ravioli and gelato.

In Mexican restaurants, select grilled fish or chicken breast, chicken fajitas, or chicken and vegetable enchiladas served with salsa. Avoid sour cream, nachos, beef burritos and guacamole.

In Japanese restaurants, choose fish or vegetable sushi, noodle dishes, steamed vegetables, tofu dishes or grilled chicken.

In Turkish or Lebanese restaurants choose bread, tabouli without dressing, vine leaves or a small serve of kebabs.

Thai restaurants are popular these days, but don't be deceived by the slender staff serving your food. Many of the menu choices contain more calories than you'd realise. If you're careful, though, you'll find some delicious low-calorie options. Try to choose steamed rice, vegetable dishes and stir-fries in a light sauce.

As you can see, there are plenty of choices that you can make, and if you're careful you can dine out at most restaurants and still sail a steady course to find the slender you.

Maintain a list of great choices

When I embarked on my weight loss journey, I steeled myself for that first Saturday morning visit to our favourite café. I ordered my coffee, but didn't order a cupcake. Magnificent valour? Not quite, but it felt like that at the time. It felt rather strange to sit there with only a drink. But I knew that I was on my way to finding the slender me, and nothing was going to stop me!

Every week after that I went back there, enjoyed my usual cup of coffee and never noticed the missing cupcake again. I tried to keep eating-out opportunities to a minimum, and when they arose I carefully selected the best choices on the menu.

Now that you know what sort of foods to choose and avoid, have a think about your favourite restaurants and cafes. You need to make some special selections whenever you dine out. Do your regular dining venues have those choices on the menu? If they don't provide the food that you can live with on your weight loss journey, you might need to choose some new eateries.

If you're going to a new restaurant, see if you can find the menu on online. You might be able to plan ahead and choose the best options before your visit.

If you once loved dining at all-you-can-eat buffets so that you could pile your plate high, you might prefer to dine somewhere else. If your friends like eating at a restaurant that serves everything with a side of French fries and no other options, then you might be able to encourage them to try somewhere new. I'm sure they'll understand how important that special journey is to you.

Never be afraid to say no when a friend, relative or colleague offers you some food that you know you shouldn't touch. Just tell them that you'd love to try some and it looks delicious, but you're on a strict diet. They'll usually understand, but if they keep pressing you, just repeat yourself. They will soon get the message.

Maintain a list of restaurants and cafes that can provide you with some great choices and make a list of the foods you'd like to choose at each venue. That way, you'll be always prepared for the challenge of eating out.

You'll be an inspiration to your friends, family and colleagues, and you can be confident that you'll finish that journey to find the slender you.

CHAPTER 18: COPING WITH ENTERTAINING

Entertaining on your weight loss journey

At times on your weight loss journey, you may face the challenge of entertaining guests. It might be a party, a dinner with friends or family, or some visitors who've come to stay for a few days. Whatever it is, you'll need to gird your loins with all your new knowledge and face the challenge head on.

Some of us don't entertain very often, so coping with that challenge won't be too difficult. Others are always entertaining because they enjoy it, or sometimes because it's a necessary part of their work or family traditions. If you entertain frequently, then you'll have much more to think about and plan for than most of us.

What does entertaining generally involve? Once, we may have brought out our favourite recipe books and cooked those delicious desserts and cakes, main courses smothered in rich sauces, and tasty high-fat savouries. We hoped that our guests would swoon at our tiramisu, praise our casseroles and want a second helping of everything we took all that time to prepare. And there we always were, right behind our guests in the queue, putting that food on our own plate and relishing every mouthful.

Now things have changed because you are on a wonderful journey to find the slender you. You love to entertain your family and friends, or you feel pressured to fulfil your social obligations. But that is not going to stop you from reaching that final destination on your weight loss journey.

How can you keep entertaining but still make sure that your journey doesn't get derailed? There are two approaches that you can take, and both work well.

Firstly, you can cook those delicious high-calorie foods that you're famous for, but eat your own special menu that complies with your healthy eating plan. If you feel emotionally pressured to keep serving your traditional dishes, then that might be the best approach.

I know that my son used to visit each week when he lived in the same city, and loved a home-cooked baked dinner and dessert. I ate diet jelly while my son and husband indulged in a dessert treat. It might be hard at first to explain to your guests why you're eating different food, and sometimes other people might pressure you because they think you're missing out or suffering. Don't listen to those arguments and if anyone is persistent then have a quiet talk to that person about the importance of your journey. Try to make them understand that you are not miserable or missing out. Instead, you are heading towards a glorious goal that will make you feel like a big winner.

The second approach that you can take is to re-think your entertaining menu and serve low-calorie dishes. You can do a complete replacement, or, if it's easier, just replace part of the menu. If you're having a buffet or platters of party food, you only need to make sure that a few items comply with your healthy eating plan. That way, you'll have something to eat and enjoy along with your guests. It won't matter if you also offer some other food for your more voracious visitors.

Both of those approaches, or a combination of the two, will see you travelling smoothly on that journey to find the slender you. You'll probably find that some of your guests will be very interested in your weight loss secrets.

A healthy menu

I'd never claim to be an excellent cook with hundreds of recipes at hand and I definitely won't be the next great television chef. But just to get you started on being the perfect host or hostess who can entertain and still lose weight, I'd like to suggest a few simple recipe and menu ideas for your next social gathering.

There are many weight loss cookery books available for some more creative options. Then you'll be fully prepared for the challenge of entertaining.

Let's start with an afternoon tea or a party where nibbles are required. You can make some healthy dips and serve them with vegetable crudités, rice crackers or bread. Healthy dips are usually made with natural yoghurt. Here are my three favourite dip recipes.

Tzatziki (Cucumber) dip

Ingredients: A large cucumber (de-seeded and chopped finely), 1-2 cups of natural yoghurt, garlic, salt and pepper for flavouring.

Combine all ingredients and chill overnight or for a few hours.

Hummus Dip

Ingredients: 600 g can chickpeas (drained), juice of 1 lemon, 100 ml of olive oil, 1 chopped garlic, salt and pepper for flavouring.

Combine all ingredients and chill overnight or for a few hours. You can vary the amount of fluid to get a good consistency.

Beetroot Dip

Ingredients: 3 fresh beetroots, juice of 1 lemon, 100 ml of olive oil, 1 cup natural yoghurt, garlic, salt and pepper for flavouring.

Trim the beetroots and spray with oil. Bake in the oven for one-and-a-half hours until cooked. Peel and chop very finely. Then combine all the ingredients and chill overnight or for a few hours. You can vary the amount of fluid to get a good consistency.

Cakes are always popular and for something sweet, try this easy-to-make cake that is healthy, high in fibre and low in calories. It also keeps well, and is surprisingly tasty.

Apricot and Sultana Loaf

Ingredients: 1 cup *All Bran* cereal, ¾ cup white sugar, ½ cup finely chopped dried apricots, ½ cup sultanas, 1¼ cups skim milk, 1½ cups self-raising flour. If desired, you can substitute other dried fruit.

Spray and line a loaf tin and pre-heat the oven to 180° C. Stir the *All Bran*, sugar and dried fruit together. Add the milk and leave in the refrigerator to soak everything for a few hours or overnight. Then add the sifted flour, gently stir and press into the loaf tin. Bake for one hour. After taking out of the oven, allow the cake to cool in the pan before inverting.

A healthy dinner party

Finally, I'd like to give you a menu idea for a low-calorie and healthy dinner party. It will keep your guests well fed and they probably won't notice that it isn't high in calories. The secret is that you should avoid adding the dressings and cream to your own meal.

Let's start with those nibbles or canapés that delight our guests before dinner. Try a healthy dip served with rice crackers, vegetables crudités and bread. Or make some little skewers of fruit and vegetables, some asparagus wrapped in bread, or thin slices of ham wrapped around a melon ball.

When your guests are seated at the dining table, start with a low-calorie vegetable soup served with some slices of bread. Or have some prawns and oysters with cocktail sauce served on the side.

For main course, barbecue some marinated skinless chicken fillets or fish. Serve that with a potato baked in its jacket and a healthy tossed salad. On the side, have some dressing for the salad and some sour cream flavoured with chives for the potato.

To finish off, you can make a delicious fresh fruit salad with any of your favourite fruits. Don't be tempted to add any sugar: you don't need it. And on the side, you can serve some whipped cream.

That is it. Your guests will go home satisfied and happy, full of praise for the wonderful meal you gave them. You will be thrilled, because you've been a wonderful host and still complied with your healthy eating plan.

There's no challenge that you can't overcome on that journey to find the slender you, and when you reach your goal you will look and feel fabulous.

CHAPTER 19: COPING WITH VACATIONS

My history with vacations and weight gain

I love any sort of vacation or mini-break, whether it's relaxing somewhere quiet, seeing some new sights or a swimming holiday. I want to enjoy every moment, and that includes those moments that involve eating.

Vacations were once a chance for me to take a break from being the chief cook at home. While away, our evening meal might be a takeaway from a fast food restaurant or a meat pie. At the seaside, we'd enjoy fish and chips.

Just a few years ago we discovered cruising. Oh dear. Delicious food was available morning, noon and night, and I took every opportunity to enjoy it. Unfortunately I gained about two kilograms on every cruise. Can you imagine what my body must have thought? It furiously added to my fat reserves ready for the big famine that was sure to be coming soon.

Unfortunately, there was no famine. All that plenty didn't stop when I returned from those cruises. After getting into the habit of overeating, I took every opportunity that presented itself to eat more than my body needed. My weight kept slowly rising like the morning sun.

I'm afraid that vacations have always been like a poisoned chalice for me because I allowed them to become a quick and easy method of gaining weight.

That changed when I began the journey to find the slender me. Several weeks into my weight loss journey, we set sail on another two-week cruise. That could have been disastrous for me, but I was desperate to ensure that it didn't sidetrack my diet.

I tried to be cautious, selecting better choices for breakfast, lunch and dinner. I ate an omelette filled with tomato, onion and mushrooms for breakfast. For lunch I chose a sandwich or a small serve of stir-fry from the Asian buffet.

Dinner proved more challenging, because we always like to eat in the main restaurant where several courses are served at the table. I tried to choose a consommé soup and some seafood for starters, and a low-calorie main course. If I wanted dessert, I asked for a scoop of sorbet. I didn't feel at all deprived, because everything was delicious.

I sometimes indulged, having a dessert at lunchtime or an extra glass of wine in the evening. I gained half a kilo, but resumed my weight loss journey as soon as I returned to the real world.

Next year I'm preparing for a longer vacation. I intend to plan more carefully and try to meet the challenge of not gaining any weight. But that will be another story, because it will be about preserving the slender me and staying slim.

Plan what to eat and drink

Vacations are an important and exciting part of life, and you should enjoy every moment of them. With some careful planning, you can go on your break and still lose weight.

The first thing to consider is the sort of vacation that you're planning. If you intend to trek in the Himalayas, take a walking tour of Tasmania's wilderness or join a cattle drive, then you probably won't derail that weight loss journey. You'll be burning plenty of calories and there won't be too many extravagant eating opportunities. Enjoy your adventurous vacation!

For anyone else, you just need to consider your vacation as a part of your weight loss journey and make some plans. Don't avoid taking a vacation and, alternatively, while you're away, don't fall into the trap of making one bad choice after another.

The best approach is to learn how to take a vacation and remain on that journey to find the slender you. So what should you do? While you're making your travel bookings and thinking about your vacation wardrobe, give some thought to the choices you'll make while you're away.

Will your vacation be self-catering, or will you be dining out? If you're taking self-catering accommodation where you can cook your own meals, try to follow your healthy eating plan as much as possible. You can choose some simple low-calorie meals that are easy to prepare. Don't forget to consider your drinking as well, and make sure that you have plenty of low-calorie drinks available. Re-read the chapters in this book about your healthy eating plan and cooking the low-fat way.

If you'll be dining out or the meals on your trip are catered, re-read the chapter on eating out. Choose low-calorie options wherever you go, and if possible attempt to avoid places that specialise in high-fat foods. Write down a list of great choices before you leave home, and make sure that you carry that list with you.

Plan your drinking as well. I know that on vacation it can be tempting to relax and have several drinks, but try to include some diet soft drinks (sodas) or water. Explain to your friends that you don't want to destroy the efforts you've already made to achieve your goals.

You'll be doing well if your weight stays steady while you're away, and even better if you lose weight. If you can maintain your motivation and make some wise choices, you'll have a wonderful time and still keep travelling on that journey to find the slender you.

Maintain your focus and motivation

What happens after you return from your vacation?

The next morning, stand on the bathroom scales. Has your weight changed? Is it higher or lower than the day before you left? Write down the result, and then set sail again on that journey of discovery to find the slender you.

Don't be discouraged if you gained weight on your vacation. You can now proceed at full speed and that weight gain will soon be a distant memory.

But has your motivation and enthusiasm decreased or disappeared while you were away?

If you feel that the dream of finding the slender you is fading, then read this book again and think about the moment of clarity when you decided to lose weight. Remember that magic pill of motivation. Somewhere deep inside your brain, try to re-discover that exciting goal and the spark of motivation that you had before you went away.

Look at your master plan and think about the slender person you want to become. Keep going on that weight loss journey, and don't look back.

CHAPTER 20: COPING WITH A DIFFICULT DAY

Everybody has those difficult days

There'll always be those difficult days when your motivation levels drop or your hunger increases and you find it challenging to stay on that weight loss journey.

Just imagine a sailor on a Panamax container ship in the middle of a voyage across the Pacific Ocean. He's had an awful day where everything seemed to go wrong. Suddenly he decides that he doesn't want to be there for a second longer. He jumps over the side of the ship and into the waters far below.

No one in a sensible frame of mind would jump off a ship in the middle of the ocean. But you may be tempted to do that many times on your journey to find the slender you. You will be enticed, almost as if you are pulled by an invisible string, to abandon ship, run for your life, head for the hills and fly the coop. Anything but stay on track for a few more hours.

We live our lives one day a time, and each morning we never know what lies ahead for that day. There's always a chance that any day might be wonderful, ordinary, dreadful or disastrous.

Sometimes we have a wonderful day when everything seems perfectly designed to make us happy. You feel elated from morning till night as you enjoy one delightful experience after another. If only life could always be like that!

Most of our lives consist of ordinary days that pass smoothly with no dramas at work and no crises at home. We stay in a positive frame of mind and enjoy any pleasures that come along.

Occasionally we have a dreadful day where everything seems to go wrong. There are mistakes and dramas at work, someone scratches your car in the car park, there's a traffic jam on the way home, one of the children gets a cold, the cat vomits and your spouse is in a bad mood. Just for a final flourish, your television won't work and your bad back is playing up.

Then there are those rare disastrous days when tragic events happen. These have a major impact on our lives and it's always wise to seek help from a medical professional or counsellor as well as the support of your friends and family when you are confronted by those difficulties.

If you have a wonderful day or a normal, pleasant, ordinary sort of day, then usually it's not too difficult to proceed on your weight loss journey and follow your healthy eating plan. Hopefully, you'll even find time to do some exercise. But if you have a dreadful day you might feel as if you're struggling to stay on the right track.

The truth is that any day, even the most wonderful of days, can become one of those difficult days on that journey to find the slender you.

On a difficult day, you might feel extra hungry and start to long for your favourite treats or extra serves of food, just to help you cope. Your motivation levels seem to vanish, and the journey ahead feels very long. You start to question your ability to stay the course and reach your final goal.

We all have those sorts of days, but if you feel that every day is a struggle then you should speak to your doctor or other qualified health professional for some advice. They're the ones best qualified to help you.

Luckily, most of us only have a difficult day occasionally and there are some great ways to help you get through it. Don't abandon ship halfway through your journey, because you'll be left behind like that sailor in the middle of the Pacific Ocean. The truth is that there will never be a better time than now to find the slender you.

The power of one day

Your job is to survive each day on that long journey to find the slender you. We live our lives one day at time, remembering the past and looking forward to the future. You don't need to worry about how to cope with your weight loss journey tomorrow. And you don't need to think about coping for another week or another month.

You'll complete the journey to find the slender you by taking one small step at a time. All you need to do is keep travelling for a single day.

My husband once looked in the wrong direction and missed walking down a flight of eight stairs. He managed to avoid falling over or hurting himself, but he took all those stairs in one giant step. It was a horrible experience that he never wants to repeat!

Your weight loss journey is like descending a flight of stairs one step at a time. You know that you'll reach the bottom of those stairs, but you need to focus on each step or you could have a nasty accident. And you can't ignore each step and try to reach the bottom in one giant leap unless you're some sort of acrobat.

We've all been up and down a wide range of staircases: wide or narrow, smooth or rough, safe or slippery. A difficult day is like taking a step on a narrow, slippery flight of stairs. You hang on tightly to the handrail and focus your thoughts and energy to make sure that you take that step safely. Can you do that for one day on your weight loss journey?

Let me share an excerpt from my diary.

Dear Diary,

Today I almost fell off the rails and off the wagon. There was morning tea at work, and I was tempted to eat a piece of delicious home-baked chocolate caramel slice. I looked, I thought, I wanted, but then I turned around and left the room just in time. It was a narrow escape.

What will happen if you have a difficult day on that weight loss journey and indulge in some calorie-laden food? Will your weight loss journey end forever? Have you wasted all the effort that you've made over the last few weeks or months?

No, of course not! If you don't follow your weight loss plan for a day or two, then read your plan again, pick yourself up and keep proceeding on that weight loss journey. Enjoy the indulgence, and don't feel guilty about it. One or two days, or even a week, will not make too much difference.

Eventually, if you keep travelling one step at a time, you'll find the slender you. We all deserve an occasional treat, but never let one day destroy all your goals. Keep taking that journey one step at a time and one day at a time.

Ways to survive a difficult day

The good news is that there are some great ways to help you survive a difficult day on your weight loss journey. It's just like being on a ship that has entered some rough waters. If you start to become seasick you can take some medication or try some trusty remedies to alleviate your symptoms. Eating green apples, dry crackers and beef soup, sucking some ginger candy or getting some fresh air can help to settle a queasy stomach.

If you have a difficult day, think about the special remedies that might help you. If you're feeling extra-hungry, try eating a low-calorie snack. If you're struggling with your motivation, think extra-hard about those wonderful goals that have made you take action to find the slender you.

Sometimes you can feel like a hungry lion ready to pounce on the first unsuspecting prey that it can find. Your body seems to be yelling and screaming that it might be a good idea to go out and seek enough food to build up your supply of fat reserves ready for the next long, cold winter. Stop right there!

It's actually good news, because you're getting to know your digestive system much better and you can recognise genuine feelings of hunger. Unfortunately, in our modern society, it's too easy to find supplies of high-calorie food that can satisfy those feelings. You know that wouldn't be a good solution to the problem of surviving that difficult day!

If you're struggling with feelings of hunger, try having a low-calorie or calorie-free snack. Look at your plan and see the great snacks that you thought might help you on a difficult day. Vegetables with hummus or salsa, rice crackers, a cup of vegetable soup or an extra piece of fruit are all delicious and won't have any impact on your journey. Now is the time to eat and enjoy them!

Sometimes, just for one day, an extra snack or a slightly larger portion size for your evening meal is all that you need to help you. You could also try having a cup of tea or coffee or a diet soft drink. Or even enjoy one glass of wine!

The other way to quell those feelings of hunger is to do some things to treat your heart, soul and mind. The list is endless, but you could meet a friend, go to a movie, see your favourite TV show or DVD, listen to some music or go for a walk. You could get a massage or facial, do a beauty treatment at home, go to an exercise class or meditate.

You could have a relaxing bath, read a book or magazine, or plan your next mini-break. Go to your nearest shopping mall and look at the fashion stores or sort through your wardrobe and put aside those clothes that are now too big for you. All of those activities will soothe your heart and mind and help to reduce your feelings of hunger.

Motivation is the special magic pill that keeps you taking action to achieve your dreams. Are struggling with your motivation on a difficult day? Spend some time to look at your goals and think about the end point of your wonderful journey.

Now is the time to sit down and re-read the plan that you created (you learn about that in a later chapter). Look at the photos of that slender person you'd like to become, and look at your weight loss calendar. Read those decreasing numbers that you entered each week. Think about how far you've already come, and that special person you want to become in the future.

Re-examine the goals and special events that that you listed in your plan. Think about each one and how wonderful you will look and feel when you find that slender person. Take a moment to look at the notes you made when you described the new you. Remember that you're getting ever closer to finding them.

Look at your favourite inspirational messages or memes. If you don't have any, try searching on the Internet or at the library! My special favourite is "nothing tastes as good as the feeling of losing weight." Repeat those messages to yourself a few times.

Talk to your friends or family and other people on a weight loss journey. Read an article about someone that has lost weight using a sane and sensible weight loss method like yours. This is not a journey you should travel all by yourself, especially on a difficult day!

There will always be difficult days on your weight loss journey. They are days when your hunger pangs increase and your motivation falls, and for a moment you might even be in danger of abandoning ship and jumping overboard. Make some good food choices to reduce your hunger, or choose a relaxing activity to soothe your body and mind. And spend some time taking a special dose of motivation, the magic pill that makes you take action to achieve your dreams.

One day you will come to the end of your weight loss journey and find the slender person you dream about.

CHAPTER 21: EVERYTHING ELSE IN YOUR LIFE

Weight loss won't solve all your problems

One day, you'll stand on those bathroom scales and realise that your weight loss journey is finished. You've found that slender person. Can it really be you in that bedroom mirror? There'll be no hiding your joy as you gaze at that incredible new person.

You deserve to feel incredibly proud and celebrate your achievement. But always remember that losing weight will not solve all of your problems or make them disappear like some sort of magic trick.

Just imagine an athlete who has won an Olympic gold medal. He's been working towards that goal and longing to fulfil his dreams for as long as he can remember. He's thrilled with his achievement as he stands on the dais and his national anthem starts to play. But does that solve all his problems? No, of course it doesn't!

The athlete still has that sore shoulder problem, concerns about his father's health and problems with his girlfriend. He doesn't have a job waiting for him at home, and he has some debts to repay.

When you find the slender you, those other problems in your life won't melt away and disappear like those excess fat reserves. Weight loss might help some of your problems, but it won't be the total solution. Those problems you might face with your mental or physical health, your career and finances or your personal relationships will still be there. Don't neglect those other aspects of your life, and don't be afraid to seek advice from any professionals who can help with your difficulties.

Your mental and physical health

On that wonderful journey to find the slender you, your extra fat reserves have disappeared. They were distributed all around your body, even in your face, neck and fingers. Those clothes you once wore now look enormous on you. The transformation in your body seems almost magical!

But there's no mystery about it, and you worked very hard to achieve your goal. The slender you will look and feel amazing and your friends will remark that you look so young and healthy. Your confidence will soar and some of your health problems will improve. You may have a lower risk of developing cancer, diabetes, blood pressure problems, heart disease and asthma. Exercise will be so much easier, and some of your aches and pains may have vanished.

But don't expect your weight loss to cure everything!

It's very important to visit your doctor before you start a weight loss program, and always take their advice about the sort of diet you should follow. Throughout your journey, make sure that your mental and physical health remains your primary concern.

Your relationships and family

Your friends and family won't change when you find the slender you, although all of your relationships may alter slightly. You'll feel like a new person who can do so much more than you did before, and you can now join in all those activities you only dreamed about before. Your friends, family and colleagues will be very proud of you and treat you a little bit like a brand new person!

Enjoy all the wonderful changes you experience. But always remember that the difficulties you face with your partner, children, other relatives or friends will still remain. You might find that your weight loss journey will give you the confidence you need to think about those issues and deal with them more effectively.

Your career and finances

Last but definitely not least, we come to the subject of money and your career. Your extra fat reserves might disappear, but that won't remove those money worries or problems with your job. You can manage without a great many things, but it's very hard to survive without money. For thousands of years humans have understood that we usually won't have financial problems if our income is more than our expenditure. When our expenditure exceeds our income, it can lead to misery.

A journey to find the slender you can make you think about other aspects of your life. You might decide to make some changes to your career path or apply for a new job. You might even decide to start your own business.

If you want to change your career, you'll need to take some concerted action to make that happen. If you have significant debt problems or a serious issue at work, you should try to find a resolution with the help of an experienced counsellor or adviser.

Always remember that the journey to find the slender you is a significant event in your life. You'll change from an overweight person to a slender one! It's so exciting that you might also decide to make some other positive changes in your life. But don't try to make too many major changes at once or you may start to become too stressed.

Consider if you need to make any changes. Seek any professional help that you need, especially if you have serious issues to deal with, and don't be afraid to admit that you need help. We can all benefit from some sensible advice.

CHAPTER 22: SEVEN DAYS OF MEAL PLANS

Options for your healthy eating plan

In Chapter Eight, I talked about a healthy eating plan and gave you an example of a daily menu. In this chapter, I'd like to give you a few more menu options, but don't feel obligated to use any of these suggestions. I'll leave you to count the calories, and also to create your own healthy, low-calorie menus.

The One Way Diet is all about you taking full control of your own healthy eating.

Here are some suggestions for a healthy breakfast

The first meal of the day is vitally important to kick-start your metabolism and give you enough energy to last all morning. Here are some breakfast ideas:

Porridge made with ⅓ cup rolled oats and a small serve of skim milk

1 slice of raisin toast with diet fruit spread or a small amount of mashed fruit

⅓ cup natural muesli and a small serve of skim milk

⅓ cup of any wholegrain cereal (check nutrition guidelines on the pack) with a small serve of skim milk

1 poached egg on 1 slice of wholemeal toast

1 slice of low-fat cheese melted on 1 slice of wholemeal toast

1 sliced tomato on 1 slice of wholemeal toast

Suggestions for a healthy lunch

By midday, your energy levels will be dropping. Here are some lunch options to get you through the afternoon:

100 g baked beans on 1 slice of wholemeal toast and a small side salad

Omelette made with 2 eggs – add mushrooms, asparagus, tomato and onion

1 slice of pitta bread, filled with 50 g lean chicken, lettuce, tomato and grated carrot

1 small bread roll filled with 50 g of salmon, lettuce and tomato.

Minestrone soup with 2 slices of rye bread and a tossed salad
2 slices of sourdough bread, 40 g pastrami and salad
Mixed green salad with a small can of mixed beans

Some suggestions for a healthy dinner

Dinner is one of the highlights of the day. Remember to pay careful attention to your serving size and always weigh meat, chicken and fish. Here are some dinner options:

Pizza made with pitta bread, prawns, fresh capsicum, tomato, onion and spices

100 g lean minute steak with mashed pumpkin, sliced carrots and broccoli

Frittata made with 2 eggs, sliced zucchini and onion

Beef casserole made with lean beef, diced vegetables and a can of tomatoes

Curried chicken salad: toss chicken cubes in 1 tablespoon of curry paste, fry and then serve on a tossed salad

100 g lean pork fillets marinated in oyster sauce, served with ¼ cup of pasta and mixed green vegetables

Low-calorie souvlaki made with 1 slice of pita bread, 1 lean lamb kebab, tomato, onion, pepper and a dressing of hummus.

As you can see, it's easy to create a wide variety of low-calorie meals that are nutritious and satisfying because they include a range of vegetables and complex carbohydrates as well as meat, chicken or fish.

CHAPTER 23: GETTING CLOSER TO YOUR GOAL

The challenge of reaching your goal

Imagine that you're an international airline pilot on a fourteen-hour flight across the Pacific from Sydney to Los Angeles. You make your preparations and do those pre-flight checks. Then you taxi the plane onto the runway and take off. That part of the flight is always the most dangerous, but you do it safely.

Once you reach cruising height, you turn on the automatic pilot and cruise for hours. But as you approach Los Angeles, you need all your skills to make the descent and safely land that plane. The biggest challenge of the flight is guiding the aircraft to the runway and touching down.

You weight loss journey is very much like that long-haul flight, and you're the pilot in control. It's a struggle at first to adhere to that healthy eating plan and change your lifestyle. That's why the initial period is so difficult. How many people do you know who stop their diet after just a few days? But you've managed to succeed and you've taken off!

As time passes, your new lifestyle becomes a habit and you see your weight loss start to fall. You achieve each mini-goal, and with the loss of every kilogram you feel motivated. You're cruising on the journey, just like that plane that cruises for hours at high altitude.

That doesn't mean that it's easy, or that there are no dangers. You need to work hard every day and keep your motivation levels high. Something could break down, you could hit turbulence, or you could head in the wrong direction. But you're prepared to deal with any difficulties that might arise. Your success so far has been amazing.

One exciting day you realise that you are getting close to your goal. You have a few more kilograms to lose. Just like that pilot, you need to bring the plane in for a safe landing. So what could go wrong now? What dangers lie ahead?

Some of you will be so highly motivated that you have no trouble heading safely towards that final goal. You're starting to look and feel almost as slender as that person you dreamed of becoming. You're receiving compliments everywhere you go, and you're fitting into smaller size clothes.

But for those very same reasons, some of you may encounter problems. You're starting to tire of that weight loss journey. You begin to ask yourself if you need to lose more weight. You already look and feel great. What more could you want? Your motivation levels start to drop. Motivation is the magic pill that makes you take action to achieve your dreams, and suddenly it is as if you're on a lower dose rate.

The other cause for trouble is a very real and physical one. You've lost weight, and when you stand in front of the mirror you're stunned at how much thinner you look. You have literally become a person with a smaller body.

A smaller car doesn't need as much petrol each day as a bigger car, and your body doesn't need as much food. It needs less fuel energy and fewer building blocks to do repairs and maintenance. Because of that, your body doesn't need as many calories each day.

To use up those final fat reserves, you need to eat less than your body needs each day. You should never drop below 1,200 calories per day (or 1,500 calories for a man). But as you get closer to your goal, that gap is narrowing.

That means your weight loss might slow down. You're not burning as many fat reserves each week because your body doesn't need them for fuel. But you're still losing weight and you'll reach your goal weight if you persevere.

Some people start to think that they're meant to be a certain weight that is above the healthy weight range for their age. They imagine that their body is trying to tell them that because their weight loss has slowed down. But unless there's a specific medical reason for your weight gain, then you know that isn't true. You can reach your goal weight.

An airline pilot needs all his skill and concentration to bring that plane in for a safe landing. You need to use the same level of skill and concentration to reach the end of your weight loss journey and find the slender you.

Revise your goals and face the challenges

That airline pilot cruises along for hours at high altitude, but he needs to work hard and think about his plans when that plane begins to descend. When you're getting close to your goal, it's time for you to have another look at your plans.

The final goal weight is listed on your plan. Is it the upper limit of the healthy weight range for your height? You're looking and feeling so much better. Do you think that your ideal weight should be several kilograms below that upper limit? If you agree, then adjust that final goal.

I certainly don't suggest that you lose much more than that. If you still feel unhappy with your body and think that you've become obsessive about your weight loss then I urge you to speak to your doctor as soon as possible.

Think about your healthy eating plan and exercise. Your weight loss might slow down because your body doesn't need to burn as many fat reserves to top up your fuel levels. But don't be tempted to drop below 1,200 calories per day (or 1,500 calories for a man). You should still lose weight if you stick to those levels of calorie consumption.

So what else could you do? First of all, re-check your eating plan and make sure that you're staying within that calorie limit. It's easy to sneak in some extra food or increase your portion sizes here and there, and before you know it your weight loss will slow to a crawl.

You could try doing a bit more exercise. An extra five or ten minutes added to your walk might give your metabolism a boost. Just try it for a few days.

Finally, think about your motivation and the four key ingredients that you need for weight loss. Has your motivation started to wane? Read your notes about the slender you and remind yourself that you can become that person.

Think about your final goal, examine your healthy eating plan and find the motivation that you need to lose those final few kilograms. You're almost there.

Head towards the slender you

That airline pilot brings the plane in for a safe landing. The plane touches down on the tarmac and the pilot makes it appear effortless, but we all know how difficult it must be. Losing those last few kilograms is never easy, but are you willing to take on the challenge and become the slender you?

I'd like to share an excerpt from my diary.

Dear Diary,

Four kilograms away from my goal weight of 60 kilograms! I'm almost shaking with excitement and can't wait to get there. Am I going to make it? I can't lower my calorie intake any more, but I can walk for an extra ten minutes a day, and maybe that will help to get me across the line.

Imagine how exhilirating it will be when you're just a few kilograms away from your goal weight! Don't give up merely because you're looking and feeling so much better. Keep travelling on that journey and believe that you'll find that slender person. Just a few more steps and a bit of extra work, and you'll be there.

CHAPTER 24: REACHING YOUR FINAL DESTINATION

Celebrate the new you

Think of what a special moment it will be. You step onto the scales and there it is: you've reached your goal weight. You've become that slender person.

That single moment when we achieve our dreams can sometimes seem almost like an anticlimax. You've done it, but there are no brass bands or fireworks. There are no crowds rising to their feet in loud applause, no jet fighters flying in formation overhead, and no twenty-one-gun salutes from the nearest rampart. But do you feel disappointed? No, of course not: because you feel wonderful!

There are people who say that losing weight won't bring you happiness. But I have yet to find a person who didn't feel hysterically, wildly happy about reaching their goal weight. The long and sometimes tedious journey is over. You feel so pleased and proud of yourself that you could shout it from the rooftop of the tallest building in town!

Take the time to enjoy that moment. Say it over and over because it will be hard to believe. You're not overweight any more. You're slender. That weight loss journey is finished, and you should feel very proud of yourself.

Now is the time to celebrate and enjoy your incredible achievement. Mark it with a vacation or a weekend away, a special dinner or even a party. Remember the occasion by buying something you want, or spending the day with someone you love. There are thousands of ways to celebrate, as long it means something very special to you.

Look at your plan to find the slender you. Make sure you write down the date, and look at those special goals you wrote down. Perhaps you wanted to lose weight for a family wedding, a holiday or another special occasion. Now you can enjoy those special events to the full, in certain knowledge that you look and feel amazing. Prepare for them and savour every moment: you deserve it!

Let me share an excerpt from my diary.

Take time to re-think your goals in life

Now that you've become that slender person, you might feel that you have a new perspective on life. You may want to tackle things you never considered possible before and re-examine your goals in life. But slow down and think carefully before you make too many dramatic changes. That can become stressful, even if they seem fun or exciting. Don't feel pressured to alter every part of your life, or make any adjustments that take you too far outside your comfort zone. For now, just focus on getting to know the new you!

Amidst the celebrations, take a moment to remember that losing weight won't solve all your problems. Difficulties and struggles that you have with your mental and physical health, your personal relationships and money will still remain.

When people are asked to consider the most important things in life, they usually mention their health and the people they love. Always remember to keep that perspective as you look to the future.

For the rest of your life you'll be on another journey – one to maintain the slender person you fought so hard to find. Don't forget that your body always tries to build up your fat reserves, and your next challenge will be to ensure that doesn't happen again. But if you can make a commitment to remain slim every single day, then you'll succeed. Always remember that you're no longer that person who over-indulges in food or drink.

Fashion, fun and the new you

You look and feel like a new person, or perhaps the same person wearing a brand new skin.

Snakes shed their outer skin regularly because they keep growing throughout their lives. Their skin becomes too tight and uncomfortable, and then they set to work rubbing against a rock. It peels off in the same way that we remove a sock, turning it inside out. Underneath is a glowing new layer of skin that is just the right size. The old skin gets left behind as the snake continues on its way.

You've managed to perform the same amazing feat as a snake! You've shed your fat reserves and uncovered the real, brand new body that now fits you perfectly. You're on top of the world!

Enjoy the all the exciting things about becoming the slender you. You've been on a long journey to discover that person, and now it's time to live life to the full.

We give so much time and energy to our families and careers that we often forget to look after ourselves. The truth is that we need to make ourselves the number priority so that we have the energy and motivation to cope with all the other demands in our busy lives.

So how can you look after yourself and enjoy that wonderful new skin of yours? First, remember to eat a healthy diet and continue doing some exercise. Now that you've found the slender you, there might be all sorts of physical activities that you want to try. Don't waste another moment of your life!

You should embrace a healthy and active lifestyle. Once, you may have been so shy that you didn't want anyone to see you going for a walk. But now you're happy to be seen doing anything that might interest you. Plan what you might like to try and get started. If you find that you don't enjoy an activity, move on to something else.

In the past, you didn't have the energy to do everything you wanted. Now you can remind yourself about all those things and start to try them one by one.

Finally, we come to the delightful topic of fashion. When you were overweight, you may have neglected your appearance and dressed in loose clothing that resembled four-man tents, or oversized shirts and trousers. Take the time to get a new hairstyle, include some personal grooming in your weekly schedule, and start to dress so that you make the most of that wonderful new figure of yours.

Whether you're a man or a woman, find the colours that suit you best and read about the latest fashions. Ask a shop assistant or a stylish friend to help you find the clothes that will flatter you the most, and tell them you don't want to look frumpy.

No matter what your age, wear clothes that drape flatteringly on your body, learn to co-ordinate your clothes well and add some accessories for an extra dash of style. If you don't have much money, shop at thrift stores or organise a swap meeting with your friends.

Try on all sorts of clothes and shoes to see how they look in that dressing room mirror. You no longer need to fear the sight of your body, and you'll be amazed at the way you look in that item you thought you couldn't possibly wear. Be brave and conquer the new world that lies before you!

You've found the slender you and you're not overweight any more. You've travelled an incredible journey and reached your goal. That makes you a very big winner! You can live your life as that slender person and feel very proud.

CHAPTER 25: FOREVER AND A DAY

My history with yo-yos

I remember watching a team of experts give a yo-yo demonstration at my primary school assembly when I was about nine years old. Those experts could walk the dog, go around the world, around the corner and rock the baby with relentless precision. All the children were enthralled and, in short, we thought they were brilliant.

The most fundamental yo-yo trick is easy to describe. The yo-yo drops down, stays for a few moments at the lowest level, and then climbs up almost as rapidly as it fell. That perfectly describes my history with weight loss and gain. Up and down, just like a yo-yo. I reached my weight loss goals, stayed for a while at that weight, and then slowly but surely my weight would rise.

I could find some photos of me over the last twenty years, shuffle them and challenge you to line them up in order. It would be a difficult task because those images would show my journey from slim to overweight then down a bit and up again with the wild abandon of a child playing with a yo-yo for the very first time.

I remember being so happy about my weight loss, and I've wondered endlessly about how I could let myself re-gain the weight I fought so hard to lose. It's as if there was a little part of my brain that turned itself off or went haywire, allowing me to make the craziest choices.

Why did it happen? My problem was that, until five years ago, I never embarked on a second journey to preserve the slender me. Now I know that after any weight loss journey it's essential to start a second journey to maintain your weight in the healthy weight range. But now I've done that for five long years and plan to stay there for the rest of my life.

Just imagine a sea captain who comes to the end of a single journey. He doesn't decide that all his work is finished forever. He knows that he needs to start preparing for a second journey very soon.

Are you prepared to face the future and preserve the slender you? Forget about the weight problems that are in your past because the story of your future will be different. If you are ready, willing and able, then you can finish your weight loss journey and then start a new journey to preserve the slender you.

A journey for the rest of your life

This is the last piece of knowledge that you need before you start to make a master plan for that journey to find the slender you. Read about it now, but then you don't need to think about it until your special journey to find the slender you is almost over. You can store it safely in the back of your mind until then.

It's like having an airline ticket to fly home after a great overseas vacation. You know that it's there, carefully secured in a safe place. But you don't worry or even think about that ticket until it's needed.

We've all heard those scary stories and statistics about the percentage of people who re-gain the weight they lose on a diet. Some people even say that losing weight isn't worth the effort, or that most diets result in failure. In an effort to solve the problem there are strange eating plans and even stranger theories designed to provide a solution. Confusing advice and mixed messages are everywhere, and it becomes hard to know what to believe.

What do people mean when they say that a diet fails? Your school and university examinations might have had a pass mark of 50%. Imagine if you passed your maths exams at school but now the records show that you failed because today you've forgotten those formulas you once memorised.

That is what some people say about diets! Many people succeed in losing weight, but when they stop their diet they re-gain that lost weight. A healthy, sensible weight loss plan will never fail to help you lose weight and achieve your goals. When people say that a diet has failed, they are only referring to the next stage of your life, that second journey of preserving the slender you.

Before you start to travel on that long weight loss journey, it's important to know that there is a way to make sure you preserve the slender you. You won't re-gain the weight you lose and you can remain slender for the rest of your life. There is a way, and it can be found deep inside your brain!

When you finish your journey to find the slender you will need to embark on a second journey to preserve the slender you and stay slim for the rest of your life. You will maintain your weight by having a healthy lifestyle and preserving the person you have become.

Don't worry about that second journey while you are travelling on your first journey to find the slender you. All you need to do is remember that when you finish your first journey there will be a second, easier journey that will last for the rest of your life. You can learn all about it after you find the slender you.

It will be like the difference between building a house and maintaining it. There is work to be done every day to keep a house in good condition, and as we know so well that work continues as long as that house keeps standing. But it's not as big a job or as difficult as that initial building process. Imagine if you had to re-build your house every week!

The truth is that you can find the slender you, and when you come to end of your weight loss journey you can stay slim for the rest of your life.

How to preserve the slender you

Is there really a strange and secret way to preserve that slender person and remain slender for the rest of your life? Before you start to plan for your future, you might like to know what lies ahead on that second journey.

Imagine the moment when you find the slender you. That long task of losing weight is finally over and you'll never want to gain another kilo. You're free to roam those fashion stores, feel fantastic and live life to the full doing all those things you could only dream of before.

But how can you preserve that slender you? Will you fall victim to the weight gain syndrome you might have experienced before or seen so many friends and relatives experience?

It's important to remember that the day you reach your goal is not a day when all your efforts are over and you can enjoy endless feasting in celebration. Your body will soon build up fat reserves if you return to excessive eating. Just think about my two-week cruises: a hearty breakfast, lunch and dinner saw me gain about a kilo a week!

You've lost your extra fat reserves and those fat reserves could return again. How can you stop that from happening?

There are two key skills that will help to prevent you gaining weight, and I think you can already guess what they will be. You'll need to follow a healthy eating plan and do some regular exercise. In other words, you will be living a healthy lifestyle!

Healthy eating and regular exercise will become an important part of your life on that journey to find the slender you. When it's time to travel on that second journey, you'll make it a major part of your normal life, and say goodbye to weight gain forever.

Have you ever dreamed of being so rich that you could live like a prince/princess or movie star? Perhaps a part of that dream was the thought of dining well and being waited on hand and foot. But the truth of the matter is that your average princess or celebrity is in the constant glare of publicity and spends a great deal of time and energy keeping fit and focused on healthy eating. If you take that second journey to preserve the slender you, then you will definitely be living the lifestyle of the rich and famous!

Will you need to follow a 1,200-calorie diet (or 1,500 calories for a man)? No, of course not! But you'll keep eating a healthy, well-balanced diet with plenty of fruits and vegetables. You'll work out the number of calories you need to *maintain* your weight and try to ensure that you generally eat that amount of food each day. And you should try to eat six times a day to keep your metabolism working and your hunger under control.

The other important part of your new lifestyle will be exercise. Make sure that regular exercise becomes an integral part of your life, and take part in any sort of physical activity that you can.

Now enough of that! You don't need to think about your second journey until you finish the first one, and the time has come to start making plans.

Just remember that when you come to end of that journey you will start a new journey to preserve the slender you by living a healthy lifestyle. That will last for the rest of your life, but you will never regret it.

CHAPTER 26: A PLAN FOR YOUR WEIGHT LOSS JOURNEY

You dreams become reality when you start to plan

You already know the first two key ingredients for weight loss. Key ingredient number one is belief: believing that you can become the slender person of your dreams. I hope that you're now determined to find that person.

You know about key ingredient number two because, after reading chapters 5 – 25, you know how to lose weight and stay on your weight loss journey until you reach the finish line.

This chapter is about the third key ingredient for weight loss. The good news is that your dream of becoming that slender person will start to become reality as soon as you begin to write your own master plan. You'll be ready to take that long and sometimes perilous journey. Your plan will help to guide you and keep you focused on reaching your final destination.

You master plan will include everything you need for that journey. You'll also have a few simple chores to do. But then you'll be ready to take action.

You've gathered all the knowledge that you need, and you believe with all your heart that you can become that slender person. That's your dream, and you know exactly what you need to do to get there. Now, at last, it's time to write a plan.

Let me share an excerpt from my diary.

Dear Diary

I'm so excited. It's exactly twelve months until my next cruise, and ten months until Christmas. How wonderful it will be to wake up on Christmas morning and know that I have the best present ever: I'm slim! I have a ten-year-old photograph of myself looking slender in a silky turquoise bathrobe, watching the children unwrap their presents. Next Christmas, I'm going to wear that again. Today, I'm writing my plan and getting ready to start my weight loss journey tomorrow.

Just imagine that you want to head off on the cruise of a lifetime. You're so excited. It's a big dream of yours, and that ship is sailing into port ready to take on passengers. But wait: you haven't made any plans yet! You've forgotten to prepare for that journey. You didn't book your cruise, you haven't cancelled the newspapers, and you haven't obtained a passport or visas. The ship is pulling away from shore and you haven't even packed your bags.

Of course, that would never happen because you would never go on a journey like that without making preparations. Your trip of a lifetime will only be a dream until you start planning.

So what do you need to do? You make the bookings, write down your itinerary, and get some travel insurance and a passport. You pack your bags and ask your neighbour to water the pot plants, collect the mail and mind the dog. When you finish planning and preparing, you'll be ready in time and everything should run smoothly.

You would never travel overseas without making sure that you'd made those plans. So why would you embark on that journey to find the slender you without making any plans? You know your final destination, and now you need to plan how you'll get there. Then you can take action and achieve your dreams.

It will only take a day or two. After designing the plan and making some preparations, you'll feel confident and ready to start that long journey.

Have you ever heard people say that the planning and anticipation of a holiday is all part of the fun? My husband doesn't always understand why I start planning my luggage for a vacation several weeks in advance, and why clothes start appearing on the clothes rack in the spare room a week or two before we leave. The truth is that I enjoy that planning, and it helps me to cope with whatever lies ahead.

Planning for your weight loss journey will definitely be fun, because you know that you're preparing for one of the best trips of your life. The plan is going to include everything you need, and it will fire you with determination to succeed. You know that you're ready to set sail, and nothing is going to stop you.

Once you get started, it will only be a matter of time until you reach your goal.

How to write your plan

You have some knowledge about weight loss and you believe that you can find the slender you. Now you're ready to write your plan, your fingers are trembling in anticipation, and your brain is in top gear. So where do you start?

Your master plan for losing weight will be the key ingredient that you need to guide you. It will include your goals, healthy eating plan, exercise, shopping and cooking, and it will record your progress. After you write your plan, there will be a few chores to do. And then you will be ready to start.

First of all, find somewhere quiet so that you can do some serious thinking. Don't rush, and don't try to do it while you're also doing ten other things at the same time. If you can't find a peaceful place at home, then go somewhere else, even to your local library or a park.

Your plan should fit on several pages, but it is entirely your decision how you format and decorate it to suit your personal taste. You might like to place it in a special folder, stick it on the wall, or just have it on the kitchen bench or in your bedroom. You can design it on the computer, or write it by hand. You can decorate it lavishly, or keep it very simple. The only rule is to include all the elements that you'll need for your weight loss journey.

Search for a photo or two (or three) that you can include. It could be a photo of yourself when you were much slimmer, or a photo of someone that you admire. It could even be a photo of some clothes that you'd like to wear when you've lost weight.

Try not to include a photo of yourself that shows you looking overweight. It will make you feel negative and discouraged. Set that aside to use as a "before" photo, but don't include it in your plan. Those days are behind you, and your master plan should be a document that makes you feel happy and excited. You've already made a great start.

Now it's time to start writing. Create or find a weekly calendar so that each week you can record your weight. As the weeks go by, you'll have a great time reading that list of decreasing numbers. Each Saturday or Sunday morning, or another convenient day, you can weigh yourself. Then you'll want to rush like a child on Christmas morning to enter the weight in your plan.

Your next task is to write down your mini-goals and include a space to enter the date you achieved them. Just imagine what you'll look and feel like when you reach each of them. The goal of finding the slender you can sometimes seem overwhelming, so you need to focus on achieving each of those mini-goals along the journey.

Re-read the chapter about mini-goals, and create your own special list. You can use five-kilogram increments of weight, and you can also use your body measurements, clothing size or anything else that has a meaning for you.

During your journey, focus on reaching the next milestone that lies ahead.

Now it's time to write down your own basic Healthy Eating Plan. That's the most important part of your plan, and the most essential element of your weight loss journey. Follow the guidelines, count the calories, and list your menu choices for breakfast, lunch, dinner and three snacks from morning till night. Don't forget to include drinks and the milk you put in your tea or coffee.

This, of course, will take you a while. Try to keep it simple and be sure to count the calories carefully. Read those chapters again about the Healthy Eating Plan, and make sure that you write a well-balanced menu with all the essential food groups and plenty of fruits and vegetables.

The next part of your plan is much more fun to think about. It's that magic pill of motivation that makes you take action to achieve your dreams. First of all, write down those special goals you're looking forward to. You'll look great on that holiday next year, or at that family wedding, or on Christmas Day. You'll be able to wear some lovely clothes, or that beautiful dress or suit that's been in your closet for a long time. Or you'll just enjoy feeling so much healthier.

Then write down all the little ways you'd like to maximise your motivation every single day. There might be things that'd you'd like to do, some low-calorie or calorie-free snacks or drinks you'd enjoy, or ways you might cope on a difficult day. Re-read the chapter on motivation and write down a few ideas. As you travel on your journey, you'll think of some more so leave space to add them.

The final thing to add to that plan is your exercise program. All you need is about thirty minutes of exercise five times a week. You don't have to think of a training program that sees you progress from a one-hundred-metre walk to running a marathon in six months. And you don't need to jog, work out at a gym or sign up for boot camp.

Make sure that your own exercise program is something that will be easy and convenient for you. As long as you're moving your body, then you're getting some exercise. If you can't manage thirty minutes, you can work slowly up to that level, starting with a few minutes each day. And if you're shy about being seen, then do your exercise at home or in your garden. Re-read that chapter on exercise and try to make it a small but enjoyable part of your life. It will help to improve both your health and your weight loss.

To finish off your plan, you can include anything else that you'd like to, including inspirational messages and a space to record your feelings. Just be sure that your plan includes your goals and mini-goals, your healthy eating plan, your exercise program and the methods you might use to motivate yourself. And make sure you have a calendar to record your weekly weight.

Your plan is finished, and now you just have some simple chores to do.

Some special chores

You've written your plan and now, so that your preparations are complete, you have some simple chores to do. Make sure you have your plan with you, because you'll need it.

First of all, you need to write a shopping list and prepare some food ready for your Healthy Eating Plan.

Just imagine one evening that you open your refrigerator and find that you've run out of your favourite no-fat fruit yoghurt. You immediately start looking for an alternative, and that might not be as low in calories. You might even be tempted to make a very bad choice. That's why your shopping list is so important. Make sure that it includes all the food in your personal healthy eating plan and everything you need to cook or prepare it.

Now you need to do some grocery shopping so that your pantry and refrigerator are the right food on hand for you, and you're prepared to cook the low-fat way. While you are out shopping, consider if you need to invest in a set of kitchen scales so that you can measure your portion sizes accurately. You might also need to buy some bathroom scales or a tape measure.

Your next chore is to sort through your pantry cupboard and refrigerator to make sure there is nothing in there that could tempt you to stray. If you can't look at the sight of a packet of chocolate cookies without getting desperate urges to open the pack and eat the lot, then throw it out or give it away. When you start to lose weight, you won't care about the loss of that food you purchased.

If you need to organise your food so that it's ready to go for your busy lifestyle, then do that now. You might want to make sandwiches or cook healthy vegetables or soups and freeze them or store them in the refrigerator. That way, you'll be prepared for your first week.

You're almost finished. There's just one more thing to do and your plans will be complete. The final task is to write down your current weight, measurements and clothing size.

If you're anything like me, you may not have weighed yourself for a long time. It takes great courage to stand on those scales for the first time in quite a while. It might be scary to see how much you weigh, or measure your waist and hips, but it's important that you write it down.

Don't be discouraged or shocked. One day, you'll be thrilled to look back and see those measurements, because it will show just how much you've lost and how far you've come on that journey. Record those measurements in your new plan and give yourself a pat on the back. Your plans and preparations are now almost complete!

How to use your plan

Now it's time to relax and perhaps you need to sleep on your plan and come back to it the next day. But if you're ready to go and as excited as a thoroughbred in the starting gate of the Melbourne Cup, then take another look at your plan right now. Are you happy with it? Does it contain everything you want to include? If you'd like to re-arrange it or make some changes, then do that now.

Look at your healthy eating plan and re-check those calories to make sure that they're accurate. Make sure you've chosen foods that you'll truly enjoy, and ones that will keep hunger at bay throughout the day. And make sure that your exercise program is not too ambitious.

The good news is that your plan is not written in stone. Once you get started, you might like to make some changes. Perhaps you'll want to modify your eating plan or exercise program.

You might think of some more motivational tools or some extra mini-goals that you want to include. And you might think of some more exciting events in the future that you'd like to have as goals. You might even decide to format or decorate your plan in a different way, or buy a special folder.

Go ahead and make all the changes that you need. During your weight loss journey, working on your plan will help to inspire and motivate you.

You've completed the plans and preparations and now you can finally take action to achieve your dreams. Use your plan to guide you. Create your menus each week, record your weekly weight and rejoice each time you enter the date when you achieve a mini-goal. This will be an exciting journey. Now you can finally take action to achieve your dreams.

CHAPTER 27: TAKE ACTION TO REACH YOUR GOAL

Now your time has come

The fourth key ingredient of weight loss is to take action, every single day, to follow your plan and achieve your goal.

Imagine that you have decided to dive from highest diving board at your local swimming pool. Full of trepidation, you climb the ladder to the top and walk out. As you get closer to the edge, the board starts to tremble under your feet. Your steps become more cautious and you stop to consider your next move.

Then, taking a breath, you peek over the edge. It's a long way down to the water, and you are terrified. Can you really do this? But you know what to expect, you've learnt how to dive, and suddenly you feel your courage rising. You brace yourself and prepare to jump.

That's where you are right now. You believe that you can become the slender you, you have all the knowledge that you need about how to find that person, and you've made your plans and preparations. You also have that wonderful magic pill of motivation, which makes you take action to achieve your goals.

So there you are, standing on the edge of that diving board. Will you jump in, or will you step back and climb sheepishly down the ladder?

You brace yourself, and in one instant you dive off that platform and into the pool below. You know that there's no turning back. Before you know it, you've plunged into the water and bounced back to the surface. You've done it!

The fourth key ingredient that you need for weight loss is action. You've turned your dream into a plan, and now you need to take action and start your weight loss journey. You can look at your plan and admire it, and you can dream and wish desperately that you could lose weight. But until you take action, it won't happen.

What's the action that you need to take? You need to implement your plan.

First of all, you need to follow your healthy eating plan.

Secondly, you need to do some exercise.

And thirdly, you need to work hard to keep your motivation levels high.

I must admit that you won't find me anywhere near a diving board. But I know that it takes just as much courage to take that first step on your weight loss journey as it does to dive into that water.

Let me share an excerpt from my diary.

Dear Diary,

I've come to the end of Day One on my journey, and I can hardly believe it. I didn't think that I could survive without a big breakfast, lunch and dinner, not to mention all those cookies. But I did it. I felt hungry, but I did it! There I was, following that diet with a small serve of porridge for breakfast, a single ham sandwich with lettuce, tomato and cucumber at lunch, a piece of fruit in the morning and afternoon, and a small, healthy dinner. I felt fine, I enjoyed every mouthful that I ate, and I'm on my way. I'm going to keep on travelling until I reach the end of my journey.

Day One of your journey is always the hardest. With such a big change to your diet, you might feel hungry and the journey ahead of you might seem unreasonably long. Remember that in a week or two your new way of life will begin to become a habit. And by then, your weight will be starting to decrease!

It's your turn now to take the first step on that journey. It's time to take action so that you can achieve your dreams and find that slender you.

You can get through Day One, and then Day Two. By eating six times a day, you won't feel hungry for long. Soon, you've finished your first week and your second week, and you know that nothing will stop you.

Follow each step of your plan

Here is a diary extract written part of the way through my weight loss journey.

Dear Diary,

Today I stood on the scales and I weighed 79.8 kilograms! At last I'm below 80 kilograms and I've reached my third mini-goal. I took out my plan, carefully entered that measurement in my weekly calendar and wrote the date beside my third mini-goal. I'm bursting with pride and happiness. To celebrate my achievement, I wandered around the shopping mall to dream of buying some new clothes in the not-too-distant future. Then I met a friend for a chat over coffee.

To find the slender you, take action and follow each step of your plan. A dive into a swimming pool is over very quickly. But a weight loss journey takes a long time, and it takes effort every single day.

That's why you need to complete your journey one step at a time, each day and each week. You need to live for today and live each day to the full, while you dream of your future.

The great news is that your journey is so rewarding. You'll be delighted every time you reach a mini-goal. Whenever you lose a kilogram, you know that you're looking and feeling just a bit better. And as you get closer to your final goal, you start to look so slender you will be amazed.

Many of us would like to drive across Australia one day, and it might be something we plan to do when we retire. But only a few hardy people have chosen to walk that distance. It's over four thousand kilometres (or two-and-a-half thousand miles) from Melbourne to Perth. Adventurers who have attempted that journey took over one hundred days to complete it.

Most of would never consider such a long and exhausting challenge that must take a terrible physical toll on the body. But just suppose there is a grandmother who wants to achieve that goal. There's no way she could walk all day, every day but she decides that it might be possible if she could walk just three kilometres a day, as long as there was some good food and a comfortable place to stay each night.

She sets off and walks for less than an hour each day, one step at a time, and finally reaches Perth. She has achieved her goal, even though it takes her three-and-a-half years.

Of course, none of us would want to spend several years walking across Australia. But most of us would be capable of trying if we could travel a very short distance each day.

The truth is that your weight loss journey can sometimes seem as long and arduous as a walk across the Nullarbor Plain. That's especially true for those with a large amount of weight to lose. But every small step you take, one after the other, will lead to that finishing line.

The wonderful thing is that the more you have to lose on that weight loss journey, the more you have to gain!

Focus on each day and the journey you're taking during the course of that day. Don't worry about how you'll cope tomorrow. Sometimes you might feel tired or discouraged, and then it's enough to focus just on the next hour or two. But if you take one step at a time you'll reach the end and find the slender you.

Remember to use all the tools that you have to help you along the way, and consider all the aspects of your plan. Think constantly about your motivation, and all those goals you long to achieve. Don't let a vacation or a meal at a restaurant derail your journey to find the slender you. And make sure that your exercise program becomes a regular part of your life.

Never forget that the most important tool for your weight loss journey is your healthy eating plan. As time passes, keep checking to make sure that you're following each aspect of that plan. You need to eat six times a day and carefully watch your calorie count. Always eat a balanced diet that satisfies your hunger all day long and gives your body all the nutrients it needs.

Each day that you take action to implement your plan will be one more step on that journey. Soon, before you know it, you'll reach your goal.

Find the slender you

One day I reached the end of my journey. I stood on the scales and there it was: 60 kilograms. Think about what a small step it is to stand on those bathroom scales, barely three centimetres above the ground, merely to look down and see that number. But it had taken months of work to get there.

Dear Diary,

Today I stood on the scales and knew that I had found the slender me. To celebrate the moment, I took that silky turquoise bathrobe from the closet and carefully slipped it on. I looked so slender that I admired myself for all of five minutes in the mirror. Was it my imagination or did I look fantastic? I've made it!

Can you imagine how thrilling it will be for you? You'll feel like a new person, and you won't be able to wipe the smile off your face. It will almost feel as if you're wearing a new skin, and you'll also breathe a sigh of relief that the long journey has come to an end.

You can walk into a store and approach the clothing racks containing small size clothes. Try them on and they'll actually fit you. People will admire your achievement and compliment you on your new appearance.

Best of all, your body will feel lighter and you'll be able to walk and run around more freely, play with your children and do those physical activities you couldn't do before. You'll feel healthier and happier, and your doctor will be very pleased with you.

Let me be the first to congratulate you when you take that initial step on day one of your weight loss journey, and when you survive your first week and then your second week. I know how difficult it can be, but it's definitely worth the effort.

Some people can never do anything more than dream about the goals they would like to achieve. But if you take action to achieve your dreams, then one day you'll succeed.

When you reach that milestone, you can tell yourself that you used the four key ingredients to help you lose weight. The first two key ingredients were that you believed that you could become the slender you, and you gained the knowledge so that you understood how to lose weight.

The third key ingredient was to make a plan to help and guide you on your weight loss journey. Finally, and most courageous of all, you used the fourth key ingredient. You took action, day after day, to achieve your dream.

To keep staying the course on that journey, you used the magic pill of motivation. That's the thought process in your brain that made you take action to achieve your goals. It's all been your own hard work and now you've become the slender you.

Take the time to celebrate and enjoy that magical moment. Enter that final result in your weight loss plan. Look at your goals and prepare to enjoy those special events you wrote down months ago. You'll look and feel great at all of them.

Pull out the "before" photograph that you placed in a drawer. Look at it carefully, and look at yourself in the mirror. How different do you look? It will depend on the amount of weight you've lost, but some of you may barely recognise that old image. You'd never want to go back to the past and be like that again.

What does the future hold for you? We can never know what lies ahead, but you can take some control of your destiny and decide that you'll stay slim forever. Take the time to read Chapter 25 once more, because it talks about your life from now on.

The truth is that you must now start another journey. The good news, though, is that the challenge of preserving the slender you will be much easier than the long journey to find that person.

I'm determined to stay slim for the rest of my life. Do you share that determination? Here's a final excerpt from my diary.

Dear Diary

I have some new clothes and I'm planning the wardrobe for my next cruise. I can look forward to the future, now that I'm no longer overweight, and feel as if I can truly live my life to the full and make the most of every day.

The journey to find the slender me is over.

Now I'm starting a new journey. For the rest of my life I want to stay slim.

THE END

A Note from the Author

Thank you so much for reading THE ONE WAY DIET. If you enjoyed it, please tell your friends and spread the word on your favourite social media sites, including Facebook, Goodreads and Twitter.

If possible, would you be able to take a moment to review this book on Amazon and share your opinion? That allows me to hear your views and also helps other potential readers.

My Amazon Author page is an easy way to access all my books, including fiction books. There are three books in *Jotham Fletcher Mystery Thriller Series*:

Book 1 - THE MAGUS COVENANT

Book 2 - THE ROCK OF MAGUS

Book 3 – THE MAGUS EPIPHANY.

You can read more about me on my website at www.tonipike.com. I would be delighted to hear from you, and please let me know if you would like to be added to my email list.

I also have a book of travel tips, HAPPY TRAVELS 101. If you would like to see some of my travel photos, here is my Instagram page: @authorlovestravel.

Yours sincerely,

Toni Pike

www.ingramcontent.com/pod-product-compliance
Lightning Source LLC
Chambersburg PA
CBHW031235250726
48655CB00005B/1963